About the Author

Penny Brohn has a degree in sociology from Leeds University and has worked in Bristol as a Child Care Officer and then as a Polytechnic lecturer. Having studied acupuncture with a Chinese doctor, she became a qualified acupuncturist. She is a co-founder of the Bristol Cancer Help Centre which was opened in 1983. Penny Brohn was involved in the making of *A Gentle Way with Cancer*, the BBC2 series about alternative ways of treating cancer and is the author of *Gentle Giants*.

Also published by Century
*Gentle Giants: The powerful story of one woman's
unconventional struggle against cancer* by Penny Brohn
(Century, 1987)
*The Bristol Recipe Book: Over 150 recipes from the Cancer
Help Kitchen* by Sadhya Rippon (Century, 1987)

THE BRISTOL PROGRAMME

An introduction to the holistic therapies
practised by the Bristol Cancer Help Centre

Penny Brohn

CENTURY

LONDON   SYDNEY   AUCKLAND   JOHANNESBURG

First published in 1987 by Century Hutchinson Ltd.,
Brookmount House, 62-65 Chandos Place, Covent Garden,
London, WC2N 4NW

Reprinted 1987, 1988, 1989 (twice), 1990

Random Century Australia (Pty) Ltd.,
20 Alfred Street, Milsons Point, Sydney, NSW 2061,
Australia

Random Century New Zealand Ltd.,
9-11 Rothwell Avenue, Albany, Auckland 10,
New Zealand

Random Century South Africa (Pty) Ltd.,
PO Box 337, Bergvlei 2012, South Africa

Filmset by Deltatype, Ellesmere Port

Printed and bound in Great Britain by
The Guernsey Press Co. Ltd., Guernsey, Channel Islands

British Library Cataloguing in Publication Data

Brohn, Penny
    The Bristol programme: an introduction
    to the holistic therapies practised by
    the Bristol Cancer Help Centre.
    1. Cancer   2. Holistic medicine
    I. Title.
    616.99′406   RC262

ISBN 0–7126–1513–X

Contents

List of Illustrations

1

An Introduction to the Bristol Centre

In the beginning:

The idea of starting the Bristol Cancer Help Centre came out of a visit that Pat Pilkington made to me when I was a patient in a cancer clinic in Germany in 1979.

As a result of being spectacularly mismanaged in hospital I had fled from England with a bruised, leaky wound in my breast, a bag of sterile dressings and the terrifying diagnosis of a carcinoma. I have told the story of this rather bizarre behaviour in my first book (*Gentle Giants*). Suffice it to say here that I finally landed up in the hands of Dr Josef Issels in his famous RingbergKlinik and this is where Pat came to see me. At the height of a raging fever (one that had been deliberately induced to stimulate and encourage my immune system to fight the cancer cells) I whimpered to Pat that if I survived long enough I would put all my wit and wisdom into starting a holistic centre for the treatment of cancer in Bristol. There had to be an easier way for people to find holistic cancer treatment than the one I had been forced to take. She readily agreed to this, perhaps because the chances of my surviving the fever, let alone the next ten years, looked none too reliable. It probably seemed rather an unlikely proposition at the time. However, with a delightful touch of Jungian synchronicity, she returned home to find a letter of introduction to Dr Alec Forbes who was interested in new ways of treating cancer. Within weeks of my return from Germany (in considerably better shape than that in which I had left) the three of us met together and decided to go ahead with the plan to start a Centre.

It is interesting that Pat brought to our meetings her

experience and understanding of spiritual healing; Alec his years of knowledge and expertise regarding the function and performance of the physical body; and myself a background in the behavioural sciences and some knowledge of the influence and effect of mind and beliefs on performance. From the very beginning we attempted to respect and serve the needs of every aspect of a person's sickness in terms of body, mind and spirit.

My dignified, if untimely, retreat from hospital was due entirely to the fact that I was aware of having cancer of the mind and soul, as well as cancer of the breast. I wanted to set up a place where people could come if they felt the same: a place where therapists would show as much interest in what was going on in their patients' heads and hearts as in their livers and lymph glands.

Our first principle, therefore, was that our Centre should be holistic.

Second only to the fear of death that the cancer diagnosis evokes is the sense of helplessness it engenders. The feeling that there is nothing you can do to help yourself allows a voodoo-like doom to settle around you that is very difficult to shake off. No amount of being told to 'be positive and optimistic' or to 'put it all behind you' can counteract the feeling that if it's happened once it might happen again. Even patients whose surgery and other treatments are so successful that no sign of the cancer remains harbour the fear that it will one day come back. If we shift the responsibility for health so that it is no longer exclusively in the doctor's hands, but allow the patient to play a part as well, we go a long way towards relieving feelings of helplessness and futility.

One of the remarks that drove me from hospital was the stubborn insistence that I could do 'nothing' to help myself recover. If I could have seen a part for me to play in the treatment of my cancer I might have stayed and let the doctors play their part as well. What Pat and Alec and I wanted to do was to show people what they could do to help themselves.

Our second principle was that patients have the right to assume some responsibility for their own health. We wanted to allow and encourage people to do this.

Even cancer patients who have been clear of all signs of the disease for years often live in fear of getting it again. The great weakness of current hospital cancer treatments is that they only get rid of the symptom. I say 'only' as if that were no mean feat – it is of course very important to relieve the body of the poisonous, destructive burden of cancer whenever possible – but, however brilliantly the surgeon excises or the radio-therapist kills the cancer cells, it is still true that only the symptom has been dealt with and not the cause.

Why some people get cancer again and again despite being 'successfully' treated is something of a mystery, but just knowing this to be the case made me feel that treatment of the symptom alone was not enough. Josef Issels' therapy was designed to treat the whole body in the attempt to make each patient an inhospitable environment for cancer. In other words to help the body become so healthy that the cancer couldn't grow there. This appealed to me very much, and Alec Forbes was of course dedicated to the idea of prevention as well as cure.

Our third principle involved the teaching and practice of a lifestyle designed to prevent cancer occurring or reoccurring.

Although it is hard for me to isolate the reasons why I felt driven away from hospital it is true that I had for many years been involved in the use of 'natural' non-toxic remedies for disease. This had led me to being slightly antagonistic towards the harsh and rather aggressive methods of treatment on offer from the conventional medical world. I do not wish to imply that these methods do not have their place in the overall treatment of cancer, but I was convinced that gentler, more subtle methods could also be effective. Alec Forbes had for years become progressively disturbed by the trend towards toxic, invasive treatments and continued to hold dear the Hippocratic oath that he should 'do no harm'. We were both keen to revive an interest in, and a better understanding of, softer and kinder ways of restoring a person to health; ways that had been swept aside or overshadowed by the high-technology revolution in twentieth-century medicine.

Our fourth guiding principle was that we would educate and inform our patients about safe and gentle therapies they could use to counteract disease and enhance health.

We expanded our circle to include nutritionists, herbalists, spiritual healers, counsellors, yoga teachers – anybody who shared our basic belief system and who wanted to help. The plan was to operate for one day a week, offering advice and guidance to six patients at a time. We put together a rota of volunteers prepared to cook, clean, answer telephones, administer healing, teach relaxation, explain, clarify, care and keep records. We never advertised our presence and we were inundated with patients from the very beginning. The role of telephonist soon became the most stressful of all the jobs because we simply could not handle the number of people who wanted to come. The waiting list grew longer and longer: on hearing we could not see them for weeks, or even months, people broke down and wept, 'I'll be dead by then!'

We increased our service from one day to two, but they still kept coming. Gaining in confidence and expertise we incorporated the help of more therapists and the self-help programme we were teaching became fuller. It was just too much to learn in one day so we expanded into three days, suggesting patients stayed overnight in nearby hotels. By this time we had stretched our volunteers beyond all reason and the poor patients were leaving exhausted at the end of a schedule that was far too busy and tiring. Knowing that the need was there, increasingly certain that we had something important and valuable to contribute to the welfare and healing of cancer patients, we borrowed an enormous sum of money and bought Grove House, our present home. Prince Charles came and opened our new premises in July 1983.

We are now able to offer a self-help programme that involves a week's training. Patients arrive and settle in on Sunday evening and stay until the following weekend. During this time they see doctors, counsellors, nutritionists, healers and other practitioners of natural medicine; they talk through their problems in private sessions and in groups; they join in classes and learn a variety of ways of coping with and controlling cancer; they learn new ways of living; they think about how they might like to die. We still offer a one-day introductory programme for people who are interested, but want to know more before committing themselves to a week with us.

The Cancer Help Centre is a charity. I was horrified at how much money it cost me to get the sort of help I needed when I was ill, and one of our aims from the beginning was to make our services available to everyone; that money – or the lack of it – should never stand in the way of people coming to us. When we first started the Centre it was staffed entirely by unpaid volunteers. Thanks to this, and the fact that the Guy Pilkington Foundation picked up all the bills, we were able to offer our services free. Since then the Charitable Company has borrowed a great deal of money and, quite properly, we are paying our staff a decent salary. In these circumstances it seemed sensible to make a charge to those people who can afford it. Unfortunately this has led to the idea that Bristol is exclusive and expensive and not freely available to everyone. Nothing could be further from the truth. Bristol is a charity and there are funds on hand to cover the costs for people who cannot afford to pay. In reality even the people who do pay are only paying a fraction of what it costs us to give the service we do. Money should never be a barrier: if you want to come to Bristol, please contact us.

Our fifth principle was that the work of the Centre should be easily available to everyone and that it should be a non-profit-making organization.

Although the programme has been adapted and modified over the years the work done at Bristol is still faithful to our original principles: we offer a holistic approach to the treatment of cancer in which the patients take responsibility for their illness and are educated in the ways of prevention.

Our continued popularity and success has been due to the fact that we are clearly meeting the needs of cancer patients that are not being adequately met in hospital. But it is also true to say that we have had some very interesting results. Some of our patients claim unequivocally that they have arrested or controlled the progress of their cancer by practising what they have learned at Bristol. This is difficult to prove in the way we are used to having things proved because although we have been carefully collecting data at Bristol over the years, we have not been in existence long enough to produce hard statistics. The time span involved is rather short for our figures to have much statistical significance but we have had some dramatic case histories that have aroused a great deal of interest. So much interest that we are currently cooperating with the Imperial Cancer Research Fund on two separate research programmes to study the survival and quality of life of patients who come to Bristol in comparison with those who do not. This means that in a few years' time we should be able to produce facts and figures to support what we believe to be true, that time spent at Bristol can have a profound effect on the performance and survival of cancer patients.

Producing protocols for research and subsequent statistics concerning holistic therapies is very difficult. This is due mainly to the problem of isolating the variables. If a person changes his diet, adopts a life of regular meditation, sees a spiritual healer regularly and then claims to get better, what is it that is improving his condition? Is it morally right for us to suggest he should drop all but one of his activities just so we can find out? This would be particularly improper if there was a synergistic effect at work; in other words that the various elements work differently in combination than in isolation. There are other difficulties to do with separating the effect of a therapy from the effect of a therapist! All these things are being looked at and gradually better methods of assessment will emerge.

In the meantime one of our doctors is currently compiling a book of detailed case histories covering the lives of some of our patients. This will make very interesting reading but it will not constitute the so-called 'scientific proof' that has become so popular in our culture. However cancer patients who are disenchanted with the limitations of hospital treatment are not prepared to wait around for years and years until the methods and approach employed at Bristol become accepted by future generations. They want to start now and I am writing this book for them.

Josef Issels stated in his book, *Cancer – A Second Opinion* (1975), and repeated to me many times: 'Cancer can never occur in a healthy body. A healthy body is in the position to recognize the cancer cells and to reject them. However the defence mechanism of the body can become damaged in many ways and will eventually lose the power of being able to reject the cancer cells.'

Bristol offers patients both the opportunity to ask why their defences became damaged and at the same time shows ways in which the wonderful self-regulating system that maintains good health in body, mind and spirit may be restored.

If Issels' view – and that of the many others who think like him – is correct, that cancer can never occur in a healthy body, then a good cancer control regime should consist of more than controlling the symptom, it should include ways of returning the body to good health. This book is not a book about 'cures', it is a book about ways of regaining health. It is about an approach to the problems of disease, pain and suffering and in some ways it is appropriate for anyone, but it has been written with the cancer patient in mind.

It is called *The Bristol Programme* because there is no one single method used at Bristol. We encourage patients to pack up their own individual parcel of processes and techniques; we help them to make sense of what they are doing; we stand by them whatever they do.

The Implications of the Holistic Model

When I wrote my first book about cancer I was primarily concerned with writing about the emotional and psychological effect the disease had on me. As far as possible I tried to concentrate on the feelings the disease aroused, both in me and the people around me. Inevitably I referred to the various treatments I had, but they were not the main subject of the book. I thought such information about therapies would distract from what I wanted to say about cancer as an existential crisis. I did not want to imply that treatments which worked for me were the 'right' ones or the 'best' ones and should therefore automatically be pursued by all cancer patients. Had I given a more detailed account of the various ways in which I tried to treat my cancer it might have led people to assume that the same things would automatically work for them.

Nothing has happened to make me change this view. In fact quite the reverse. My experience over the years has led me more and more towards the belief that both the initial cause and subsequent control of cancer are likely to be highly personal experiences. This means that details of one person's individual recovery are of limited value. Not that books written along these lines don't make terrific reading, and if we're looking for inspiration then these sagas are well worth while, but if it is information we are after then we should be wary. I avoided writing a prescriptive book about my personal cancer control programme and it is not my intention to write a prescriptive book about Bristol either. This is because I share with my colleagues at the Centre the belief that our attitude to, and treatment of, disease should be holistic. This approach does not lend itself to prescriptive writing.

The word 'holistic' or 'wholistic' has come to be associated with alternative therapies but it is not a concept exclusive to any one branch of medicine or healing. It depends as much on the attitude of the practitioner as on a particular method or technique. The word comes from the Greek word meaning 'the whole' and implies that everything is being taken into account. If our nervous confession to having haemorrhoids is swept airily to one side by the specialist we are consulting about our tennis elbow, then we are not being treated holistically. Indeed the very word 'specialist' is indicative of a tendency to move away from seeing the patient as a whole towards a style of studying him in small, identifiable parts. People are increasingly fed up with being compartmentalized in this way, and, perhaps because of this, more and more doctors are making a conscious effort to see each patient as a whole – at least physically. At the level of the general practitioner certainly it is reasonable to expect that if your doctor is treating you for migraine he or she is likely to take account of the fact that you are also diabetic or had a baby two weeks ago. Some of us are more fortunate than others in this respect, but these are still only examples of the holistic principle being applied at the level of the physical body alone.

One thing that emerges frequently when talking to cancer patients is that, while their physical body comes in for a lot of medical attention in terms of examination and treatment, the person housed in that body is virtually ignored. This is all the more unsatisfactory because at the time of diagnosis the vast majority of cancer patients suffer more mentally than they do physically. Some patients maintain that this is still true after many years of struggling with the disease. Despite general agreement about this from doctors and patients alike, the hospital system is still geared towards the need of the physical body.

Like many others I found myself making demands on the hospital system and staff that they simply could not meet. I can see the silly side of this now, but it felt dreadful at the time. I remember saying to an eager-faced young doctor, 'I'm not just having a lump in my breast – I'm having an Existential Crisis.' I can see him now, so surprised he was rendered speechless, only able to stumble backwards through the curtains round my bed in order to get away from me as quickly as possible. What else could he do? Nobody had taught him about 'existential crisis' in medical school, he'd never had one of his own, and he certainly didn't want to take mine on. I don't blame him either, but it was only clear to me later that I was looking for help in the wrong place. Because of the influence of the dreadful Cartesian body/mind split in the development of current medical thinking we are training doctors who might (if you're lucky) take a holistic view of the physical body, but who are likely to ignore, or do very little about, the emotional, mental and spiritual suffering of their patients. Until we start training our doctors differently those of us who want a truly holistic view of our cancer problem will have to shop around to find it.

Bristol would be a good place to start looking. We do not concentrate only on the effect of the manifestation of cancer on the physical body. We encourage patients to look at the influence the disease has on their feelings, their emotions, their beliefs and so on. The Bristol staff all have their own specialities and bring different experiences and healing systems into the Centre, but they are all united in the attempt to work to a holistic model. They are trying to see each individual who comes there in body, mind and spirit, and they encourage patients to look at themselves in this way too.

This is a refreshing departure from the habit some hospitals have of referring to patients as cases. I was myself once greeted with a breezy cry of: 'Now what have we here? Ah, a grade one carcinoma of the left breast.' Perhaps worse even than that was the experience of an acquaintance of mine who was introduced by her oncologist to his assistant as 'the interesting liver secondary I told you about'. In all fairness it must be said that there are hundreds of hospital personnel who would never dream of doing such a thing, but in a system which attaches so much importance to the classification of disease according to symptoms, then it would be an easy mistake to make. At Bristol we are trying to take a broad overview of everything that is going on for each person we see. This means we never end up with categories, we simply acquire an ever-increasing number of unique, individual people. As a result of looking at each patient as unique, with special and personal aspects that make him different from anybody else, then we should, ideally, end up with a cancer control programme that is tailored to his requirements and nobody else's. This means that writing a book about the Bristol approach to cancer presents the same kind of challenge as my attempts at writing about my personal experiences with it.

There is not one single way of dealing with cancer that works successfully for everyone. If that were so I would not be writing this book and you would not be reading it. We all know people who have listened to a good prognosis from their oncologist, faithfully and bravely undergone a string of specified therapies, been sent home with optimistic phrases ringing in their ears – 'you're completely clear now, just forget all about it' – only to find the cancer creeping up on them again at a later date. We can set against this knowledge the fact that there are people who do make a full recovery, live a long life and die of something else. This only tells us that sometimes symptomatic, interventionist, high-technology cancer treatments work for some people but not for others.

I have met people who have claimed that they received no conventional treatment at all but by putting themselves on a special diet, or pursuing some bizarre alternative therapy overcame cancer by themselves. I have also met lots of people who have tried the same methods to no avail. This only tells us that gentler, self-generated healing methods work for some people but not for others.

At the end of the day we are left with a plethora of so-called cancer cures which might or might not be worth trying. It is difficult for patient and therapist alike to establish with certainty just what is needed for each individual person, but this is precisely what we need to do. The attempt to do this leads not only to a situation where each person's programme may be slightly different, but also towards the use of several different remedies at once. Of course, dealing with so many variables is not going to be neat and tidy but it creates a dynamic that I believe may be very important. It is possible that some remedies used in combination create something bigger than we might have predicted. There may be a synergistic relationship between various therapies that we shall never discover if we persist with the current passion for researching everything independently.

What we have tried to do at Bristol is to gather together information about as many ways as possible of dealing with cancer. We then advise and guide people towards finding a combination of things that will work best for them. Some people will try to adopt everything that they learn at Bristol and faithfully adhere to a busy schedule of multiple therapies for years. Other people have an intuitive feeling that they need to pursue one particular aspect of the programme, and they may do this at the expense of other suggestions. There is a good deal of flexibility and adaptability in the way we work. There has to be, because we are dealing with a dynamic model of disease that is constantly changing. It is important that we understand there are no rigid rules that everyone has to follow: there is only the right way for each particular person. You.

The idea of doing something to help oneself is very attractive to begin with, but it can lead us into difficulties. If we are not very careful, what starts out as something positive and inspiring ends up as a guilty sense of failure. I have met many people for whom the scenario goes something like this: they read a book written by someone who claims to have dissolved their cancer by going on a grape fast, and they decide to do the same. The trouble is they feel so ill and awful eating nothing but grapes (not 'sparkling-and-never-so-full-of-life' like the person in the book) that they give up this regime and promptly feel a failure. A guilty failure at that. Unfortunately many of the people who come to Bristol get caught in this trap as well. However hard the therapists try to reassure patients that they are not expected to measure up to some kind of standard against which they will be judged, sometimes people react as if they were. It would be wrong for anyone reading this book to feel that they must, should or ought to adopt any of its contents. These moral prescriptives often lead to self-judgement later. There seems to be a guilty little person inside all of us ready to be blamed for failure: perhaps this is a hangover from childhood. We should be on the look-out for this and resist feelings of guilt, blame or shame. Nobody is going to criticize your performance and there is no need for you to do so either.

Taking some responsibility for one's own health is a mature and sensible act and we should try to leave childlike feelings of failure out of the picture. I am constantly assaulted by advice from people telling me I would make a better job of healing myself if I would only do this, that or the other. They may well be right, but the point is I am doing the best I can. That is what you will do, it's all that anybody can do. We should never be ashamed of this. Instead of sticking in the role of patient, we are now trying to be our own healer as well and this requires different attitudes and responses from us.

Finally, may I make an apology and a very important point. I am sorry to be using the word 'patient' to describe people with cancer. After experimenting with various alternatives like 'client' I have come to the conclusion that deliberately avoiding the word patient has the effect of making what I write sound coy and contrived, and I want it to be quite the opposite. However, it is the most dreadful word. Don't be a 'patient'! There is an increasing amount of evidence to suggest that people who adapt and accept and generally behave in a patient fashion have the worst recovery rate of all. It has been said that 'difficult patients do best'. One of the most important things that we must do if we have cancer is to shift out of the role of the helpless victim and start taking positive action. This will require from us rather more assertive and imaginative behaviour than is traditionally expected from a patient. The transference of an adjective into a noun in this way is a fascinating bit of sociological semantics, but it is not in your interests to be a patient. I am sorry I have had to use the word at all.

What does Bristol have to offer?

Before starting on this it would be just as well to say what *not* to expect from Bristol. The Centre is not a hospital or a clinic. We do not have the facilities to serve the needs of very sick patients on our premises, so if you are very weak and ill it would be best to try some of the ideas expressed in the book, perhaps send off for the tape that goes with it, get a little bit stronger, and then make a visit. We do have doctors and nurses on hand at the Centre, but it is primarily an educational centre, not a treatment centre. It follows from this that you will not find us using any of the conventional cancer treatments.

Currently there are three main assaults made on the manifestation of cancer: surgery, radiotherapy and chemotherapy. We expect our doctors to be familiar with these treatments and able to answer patients' questions about them, but they are not available at Bristol. There are two reasons for this.

First, any attempt on our part to reproduce these treatments would be surplus to requirements. This country is well served with hospitals and out-patient departments and I have never yet heard of a patient who needed these treatments and could not get them. During a recent trip to Scandinavia I heard doctors talking about a dire shortage of therapists and equipment resulting in long waits for cancer patients needing urgent treatment. So far our National Health Service seems to be holding up under the strain of ruthless cuts and it would make no sense for us to try to reproduce at Bristol a system that has been refined to a high level of sophistication by hospital specialists for so many years.

Secondly, any attempt to treat patients in this way would distract us from concentrating on other aspects of the cancer crisis, the psychological, emotional and spiritual needs of the patient that have been neglected for so long. We prefer to put all our energies into building up that aspect of the therapeutic process.

There is no conflict between following the Bristol routines and taking conventional cancer therapy.

Most of the patients who come to Bristol have either had or are currently receiving one or more of these hospital treatments. From our observations it would seem that our patients tolerate these treatments better and suffer fewer physical and mental side-effects from them. Unfortunately many people do not know what to expect from hospital treatment and do not understand the short, inadequate explanations given by hospital staff. For that reason alone it is worth giving a word or two of explanation about what the average cancer patient might expect.

Surgery

There is something very attractive about the idea of neatly and cleanly removing cancer from the body, like scooping out the bad bit of an apple. I certainly know people who were operated on for cancer many, many years ago, before radio-therapy and chemotherapy became part of the scene, and they have survived to this day in apparently perfect health. In the absence of any other treatment one must assume that the surgery was one hundred per cent effective.

Of course, it doesn't always work like that. Sometimes it is only possible to remove part of the tumour, or it may be that the tumour is enmeshed with, or so deeply attached to, other parts of the body that it is deemed inoperable. It is also true that in some cases it is far from clear just how much tissue should be removed. Breast cancer is the best example of this. Once surgeons did what was known as a radical mastectomy, which involved the removal of the breast, a good deal of surrounding muscle, and glands from the axilla. Perhaps prompted in part by compassion they then experiemented with the removal of the breast only – this was called a simple mastectomy. Since the survival rates showed no change the more daring surgeons tried removing only the tumour, leaving the rest of the breast intact. This is known as a lumpectomy. This is usually followed up with radiotherapy as well. It soon became clear that this was just as effective as a mastectomy. These findings have been backed up by subsequent trials, so it is worth pushing your consultant a bit if you feel he is going to operate more extensively than you would like. There is a rising amount of evidence to show that surgery does not influence the survival of breast cancer patients, only local recurrence of the disease (S. W. H. Atkins, *BMJ*, vol 2, 1972.) It is now quite reasonable to ask if your operation is really necessary.

Reasonable it may be, but doctors are certainly not used to being questioned in this way. I accept that it is not easy to challenge the solution proffered by a strong, confident consultant when you are feeling weak and helpless. It is a good idea to have a friend or relative with you if you decide to open up a discussion. If you feel you might be a victim of your surgeon's own particular style or preference, then ask for a second opinion.

Remember also, that you do not have to agree to an operation and a biopsy at the same time. A biopsy is the removal of some tissue for examination in the pathology laboratory. This establishes whether the cells are malignant or benign – in other words whether you have cancer or not. For many women with suspicious lumps in the breast this procedure has taken place while they lay in an operating theatre under anaesthetic, thus allowing the surgeon to proceed at once with more extensive surgery if the results came back as cancer positive. Although on the face of it this sounds sensible because it saves time and means the patient only has to have one anaesthetic, the psychological pressure is awesome. There may be circumstances where this is the only sensible way to proceed, particularly in the case of tumours which are not easily accessible. However, where tumours are relatively superficial – breast cancer is a good example – it is possible to do a biopsy without great difficulty or heavy anaesthetic. In these circumstances choices about further surgery can be made later while the patient is awake and aware and able to play a part in the decision-making process.

Fortunately there are fewer hazards associated with surgery than ever before. The anaesthetics are being refined and improved all the time and it is usually possible to control very effectively the pain and discomfort that may follow surgical incisions. However, people are often very frightened about operations for cancer because they are afraid that the interference will cause the cancer to spread. There is some basis for this fear because the very act of repairing tissue during the formation of scars after surgery necessitates the proliferation of new cells at the site of the tumour that are especially vulnerable to becoming cancerous. It is also true that cancer cells set loose in the course of surgery may be distributed to other parts of the body and set up new sites there. However, when cancer occurs after surgery it is more likely to be a manifestation of trouble that had been present all alone.

The word 'primary' refers to the first bundle of cancer cells that grows in the body. 'Secondary' refers to other aggregations of cells that cause tumours of a similar kind at a different place all together. It may be many years after the discovery of the primary tumours that secondaries are discovered, if they develop at all. Some people only have to face the cancer crisis once in their lives and never get it again. But many patients do get secondary tumours, or they may develop what is called 'metastases'. This is the word used to describe the situation when there are many cancer sites or growths all over the body.

When cancer recurs after surgery it is hard for anyone to say whether the operation stirred things up in such a way as to encourage the distribution of cells throughout the body, or whether there were already cancer cells beginning to grow in these other places before the surgeon interfered with the primary tumour. Either situation is extremely worrying for the patient. While we still harbour the idea that, unless every single cancer cell is removed from the body, we will get it again, then we shall lead a very uneasy life. Although we know from scientific studies that it is not always necessary to remove or sterilize every cell in a malignant growth in order to effect a cure, success depends on the body's capacity to do its own 'mopping up'. The only release from anxiety about this comes from the use of therapies or techniques designed to enhance our own healing processes. If we feel we are re-awakening our own capacity to destroy cancer cells we feel a lot less upset by the thought that there might still be a few floating about.

When I departed from hospital to Issels' clinic in Germany I was in the worst possible shape surgically. An attempt had been made to remove a lump from my breast under a local anaesthetic. Nobody believed that the lump was malignant, so when it proved difficult to remove, there was no great anxiety about leaving some of it behind. It proved to be a tricky little operation and resulted in a lot of bruising and bleeding. This necessitated my staying a few nights in hospital, although the original plan had been for me to leave the same day. When the pathology report came back as cancer positive there was considerable panic and excitement. It was generally felt that I was now a high risk for metastatic spread and I was booked to have a mastectomy within days.

I have already described in *Gentle Giants* how I took this

leaky mess to Germany and how well it resolved under Issel's care. Before I went I had an important discussion with my consultant in which I asked him how long I could afford to be away, refusing his treatment, before my situation became much more serious. In other words, before the cancer spread to my axilla or anywhere else. His answer to this was, 'I think you'll be all right for a month, perhaps two, but you'll be in real trouble by Christmas.' This was in September 1979.

In point of fact I was not in any kind of trouble by that Christmas, or the following one, or the one after that. I put this down to the fact that I was receiving therapy that was designed to stimulate my own capacity to conquer cancer cells, and it worked. The hospital in England told me that my surgery had been inadequate and incomplete, but I still pulled through. I am explaining this in detail because I often meet people who are frantic with worry because they know they have cancers which are inoperable or only partially operable. I want to reassure them. Very few forms of cancer spread like a forest fire and it *is* possible for cancer to be present in the body and the body to be in control of it.

Radiotherapy

Surgery gets rid of cancer by cutting it out; radiotherapy does it by preventing cells from dividing. It is one of the great medical paradoxes of our time that cancer, which is known to be caused by exposure to X-rays, is treated by them.

As I write this I am following the chilling account of the accident at the Chernobyl nuclear power station. There is much talk of the cancer risk to future generations from the effect of radiation fall-out. We know only too well from information gathered after Hiroshima and Nagasaki what this can mean. Radiation disrupts the capacity of cells to reproduce normally. It can have disastrous effects on glands that are vital for our healthy survival, the thyroid being particularly vulnerable – hence the distribution of iodine to children.

We can see how potentially dangerous radiotherapy is when

we watch the person who is doing a routine X-ray of a broken finger put on a lead apron and scuttle behind a special screen in order to avoid an accidental dose – a dose that would be minute by the standards of the radiotherapy department. Personnel working within these departments wear dosemeter 'film badges' to indicate how much exposure they have had to damaging rays. The absolute maximum limit for a designated worker is about 5–7 rems over a year. A horrified doctor at the scene of the Chernobyl disaster has exclaimed that some of the population there have been exposed to 800 rems of radiation which he described as 'extraordinarily' dangerous. It would not be unusual for cancer patients to be treated with literally thousands of rems in the space of a few weeks.

The miracle is that this ever cures anybody, but, in fairness, it does. Just as there are people alive and well today thanks to the skill of their surgeon, so too there are people who have made impressive recoveries from cancer treated by radio-therapy. There is a big difference between doses of radio-therapy that are being picked up indiscriminately, by the whole body, and doses that are aimed very specifically at one particular part. Radiotherapy departments are full of com-puters and scientists whose job it is to locate tumours with great accuracy so that the radiotherapists will treat only the diseased part.

Treatment of this sort can have considerable benefits for patients. This is particularly noticeable when tumours have broken through the skin. They may be fungating and causing considerable misery and discomfort. Used as a palliative radiotherapy can make a great difference to this condition. But, and this is a big but, when used as a treatment to prevent recurrence of the disease, the long-term effects of radiotherapy may not be so impressive. Reports from around the world show some agreement about survival in the short term, but not in the long term (J. Stjernsward, *The Lancet*, vol 2, 1974). This may be due to the fact that the doses given vary alarmingly from one hospital to another.

Just as it may be in your interests to check up on how much surgery is really necessary for you, it would be interesting to compare in detail the amount of radiotherapy different consultants might recommend. I actually travelled half way round the world clutching a bit of paper bearing the number of rads and the intended duration in order to get a second opinion. This was necessitated by the appearance of another lump in my breast four years after the first. Since I was quite certain I knew how I had allowed this to happen, I more or less repeated my previous performance: told the hospital I would see what I could do first, and come back to them later.

Luckily for me I fell into the hands of one of the most lovely doctors ever to walk a hospital corridor: a radiotherapy oncologist whose advice was that I should have radiotherapy treatment, but who respected my wish not to comply with this. He has kindly monitored my progress for the last three years and my radiotherapy treatment has progressed no further than a crumpled piece of paper. In other words, by dragging my feet and stalling long enough to get my self-help show on the road again, I have managed not to have radiotherapy treatment.

Yet.

Radiotherapy has its place in the treatment of the cancer patient. I have seen many Bristol patients gain great relief from suffering due to the judicious and sensitive use of radiotherapy, to bone secondaries in particular. Until we find gentler, less aggressive ways of treating cancer we must accept that radiotherapy is part of the whole. As such it may be reasonable and prudent to include it alongside surgery and chemotherapy as part of a 'holistic' approach.

Although my colleagues at Bristol would agree with this, I am aware that some of my colleagues in the alternative therapy world would cheerfully have me shot at dawn for such heresy. In all the messianic excitement that has accompanied the exponential rise in the use of natural, alternative medicine there has been a tendency for exponents of these methods to reject and deride the whole drug-orientated allopathic thrust. I can quite easily see how this would happen. I have a great deal of sympathy for the homoeopath who is trying to treat a patient with a microscopic potency that is a sensitive and vulnerable substance, while at the same time the doctor is filling him with steroids. This is a very frustrating and unsatisfactory situation, but, unless we try to harmonize the many and various medical models and work together, the situation will only get worse. If we insist that one system is entirely right and another entirely wrong then we shall continue throwing stones at each other over the wall instead of building the new Jerusalem. No doubt we all have part of the truth. We must share the pieces of the jigsaw and unite in putting them together to form the whole picture, however challenging that may be.

Chemotherapy

As the word suggests, chemotherapy involves the use of various chemical compounds to poison the cancer cells. It is sometimes referred to as cytotoxic treatment because the substances used are toxic and, unfortunately, may be harmful to healthy cells as well. Basically the drugs used are ones which control growth in the cells and therefore cells that are dividing rapidly are especially vulnerable. This is good in that cancer cells are dividing rapidly, but bad in that some healthy cells have this characteristic too. Those of the scalp, digestive tract and bone marrow may also be affected by cytotoxic drugs. This is why treatment of this kind may result in unpleasant side-effects. Some patients lose their hair during treatment. Although this will almost certainly grow again it can be a very distressing experience. Other possible side-effects include nausea, vomiting, diarrhoea or constipation, headaches and loss of appetite. Much depends on the type and quantity of chemicals used and the status of the patient's general health before treatment. Not everybody suffers badly with side-effects, but it is always best to be prepared for this by discussing the situation with the doctor in charge. Many patients have said to me that they thought the side-effects of chemotherapy were sinister manifestations of further progress of their cancer and not just a natural consequence of the treatment. Obviously this would make the situation a lot harder to cope with. But telling patients what might happen may encourage them to believe that it will, so even open and frank discussion has its disadvantages.

The drugs are administered by mouth in tablet form, or by injection. Sometimes they are dripped slowly into an artery. Chemotherapy has a particularly impressive record in the treatment of leukaemia and Hodgkins's disease where wonderful recoveries are often seen.

Where does Bristol fit into all this?

It is very hard to feel positive and optimistic if someone is pouring a measured amount of toxic chemicals into your body. It is equally difficult to imagine that what goes on in a lead-lined vault behind a door saying 'Danger – Keep Out' can do you anything but harm. And who doesn't contemplate the many things that could go wrong while they lie in their operation gown waiting for the pre-med to take effect?

Bristol can help you get the most out of your hospital treatment.

As if you didn't have enough worries of your own, your head is also full of all the old wives' tales and hospital horror stories with which one's friends and relatives are so free when they hear of your plight. To add to all this, you are vaguely aware that you should be as relaxed as possible, so you now feel guilty as well because you feel anything but relaxed. Turmoil.

The relaxation, meditation and visualization methods taught at Bristol can be put to good use in these circumstances. By adopting one of these techniques we can choose whether to detach from the situation and depart into a different mental space, or whether to enter into it and turn it into a positive, healing experience.

One of our patients used a positive visualization technique to protect herself from the possibility of burning during radiotherapy treatment. She had not at this time been to Bristol, but she had read about a patient who had avoided burning by using positive visualization. Although she had not had any special training in these techniques, she decided to try it herself. When she finally came to Bristol she told us that the radiotherapist had been amazed, not just by the absence of burning, but by the almost total lack of any local reaction to the treatment.

The most famous and widely used way of using the mind to enhance tolerance of, and recovery from, heavy medical procedures is to visualize the process as having a healing and therapeutic effect. People do this in many different ways. Imagining that your white cells are sharks eating up a cauliflower, which is the tumour, is a method that has been made famous by the Simontons in their book *Getting Well Again*, but there are many, many more. One patient told me she used to picture the chemotherapy as a champagne of white light that smothered out all traces of unwanted cells. Any image that is positive and pleasant can be effective. It stands to reason that the whole experience of having potentially dangerous and frightening treatment will be less stressful if we are imagining it doing us good, than if we are shaking with fear, thinking only of the damage it might be doing.

A visit to Bristol would help to establish what are the best healing images for you. Some people work well with simple images like light, imagining their cancer cells drying and withering in the sun. Other people make better progress with more aggressive images. The important thing is to arrive at an image that feels powerful. Sometimes patients end up with quite idiosyncratic and complicated senarios. One such was a woman who used to visualize a golden Hoover buzzing around her body sucking up all the rubbish that shouldn't be there. There are no rules. Doctors and counsellors at the Centre try to encourage patients to find their own special image and work with that.

If you are reading this in despair because you are too ill to come to Bristol but have to face up to lots of tough treatment in the near future you could send for the tape that accompanies this book. We have recorded some thoughts and suggestions that might be helpful. This is based on what we have learned from our experience over the years and will be a powerful start for you. You can always learn your own special method later. Listening to this through personal headphones is particularly effective because it cuts you off from all the other noise and comment that is going on around you. It requires a special kind of confidence to remain oblivious to the conversation of hospital staff. Even the most innocent and casual-sounding remarks, like 'This wretched thing is stuck again' or 'We really need a new one of these' or 'Blast! That's what comes of government cut-backs', can strike a chill into the heart when we are already feeling scared and vulnerable. If you are listening to a voice through your tape-recorder that is taking you on a healing journey you will also miss any casual chat that might make you nervous.

Bristol may teach you how to avoid unnecessary side-effects from cancer treatments.

Surgery, radiotherapy and chemotherapy, in varying degrees, deplete the body of its vitamin and mineral resources. Professor Calman in Glasgow experimented with the use of vitamins A and C and found that their use improved the performance of his patients. Our experience at Bristol is that patients on our diet and taking the recommended supplements seem to withstand the destructive effects of cancer treatment much better. We have been able to talk to patients who know how they reacted to these treatments before coming to Bristol, and compare this with how they respond to treatment while they are on the Bristol programme. This is all very positive and encouraging since most of the people who come to Bristol are involved with conventional therapies to a greater or lesser degree. Most, but not all.

Bristol can help when there is no other help available.

I remember vividly the day that my father-in-law was told by his hospital consultant, 'I'm afraid there's nothing more that I can do for you.' Because there is a limit to how much radiotherapy and chemotherapy the body can stand, many cancer specialists come to the end of what they can safely do by way of treatment long before the patient dies. This leaves patients in the most tragic position, knowing beyond all doubt how very serious the situation is and, worse than that, knowing that the doctor cannot help when needed most.

This situation is very challenging and difficult for the doctor too. He is struggling with feelings of failure that he does not deserve, and often becomes acutely aware of how limited his personal resources are when he has nothing left to do but fall back on himself as a source of comfort and healing for the patient. Few doctors are specifically trained in ways of handling this situation, and the outcome for the patient depends very much on luck. Some doctors have developed emotionally and spiritually to the point where they can continue to minister usefully to their patient in non-medical ways, but for the vast majority of patients this is the end of the line.

At Bristol we believe there is always something that can be done to help. Counselling can help with the fear of dying; spiritual healing can prepare the way for a peaceful transition from this world; relaxation, meditation and visualization can help with pain control; and the diet and supplements help to raise energy levels.

I am often asked how Bristol differs from a hospice for these patients, and of course in some respects there are similarities, but there is one very great difference. People usually go to a hospice when they are expected to die quite soon. Many of the patients who can no longer have conventional cancer treatment may live for a very long time. The Bristol methods will help them to achieve the best quality of life possible during that time. We are very fortunate in this country that the hospice movement enables people to be nursed with such skill and sensitivity at the very end of their lives. Bristol is not able to offer this facility, but we often watch our patients living active lives with their cancer for months or even years.

Many of our patients report to us that their consultants are surprised to see them looking and feeling as well as they do. Very often the person doesn't match up with the patient. By this I mean that the results of CAT scans and the evidence of blood tests lead the doctor to assume the patient will be in much poorer shape than they find him. Evidently the self-help programme is having some effect.

The only other circumstances when Bristol offers something independently of the hospital regimen is when patients refuse conventional therapy. This is a particularly sensitive area. I know from my discussions with doctors that many of them are under the impression that the Bristol staff discourage patients from accepting orthodox treatment. This is most categorically *not* the case. It is a good example of the polarization that occurs when there is insufficient dialogue between different groups of people. This is such a touchy area that we actually ask patients to sign a document when they come to us in which they declare that they are not being encouraged in any way to spurn any other therapy.

No doubt the idea that Bristol has set itself up as a radical alternative to conventional therapy came about partly because I myself have refused to comply with orthodoxy on several occasions, and the media have made much of this. However I am not myself a Bristol patient, and I am not typical of the people who come to us. Even so, we do have people coming to us on occasions who are adamant about refusing conventional treatment and we would not turn such a person away.

It would interest many hospital doctors to know that there have been times when our medical team have expressed great concern to me about patients bluntly refusing hospital treatment that our doctors felt they would benefit from having. In these circumstances we can only advise and guide, we would never put a patient under pressure and force them to do something against which they have such strong resistance. It is understandable that so long as there are patients who use Bristol as an alternative, then consultants will conclude that this is how we present ourselves to them. This is not the case, as doctors who have visited the Centre know and understand. However we would continue to do all we can for a patient who is refusing conventional therapy and consequently we do have a very small percentage of patients who use only the Bristol techniques. This number is too small to produce significant statistics. Naturally some of these people have not conquered their disease and have subsequently died. But some have survived and now consider themselves to be completely free of cancer.

One lady came to us with the determination not to have any more conventional treatment. She had found a lump in her breast and was advised to have a mastectomy. She refused this and had only the lump removed. However another, bigger, lump grew quite quickly in the same breast and she was recommended again to have the whole breast removed. Again she refused. She put herself on a grape fast and came to Bristol. Within a year her tumour had disappeared. This was confirmed by her doctor and surgeon and there has been no sign of disease since. Because she has put all her faith in gentler therapy, and her good health is attributable only to these methods, she is an inspiration to patients.

If people are absolutely determined in their resolve not to have conventional treatment then they need more help than almost anybody else. For them Bristol is an alternative. For others our methods are used alongside hospital treatments in a complementary way, or they are adopted when hospitals can do no more. Whatever the circumstances, the Bristol methods have one great advantage over most cancer treatments: they are safe. True to our original principles we teach therapies that will do no harm.

The Centre has been described in many different ways over the years. The programme has been dismissed as a lot of harmless and cranky advice, at one end of the scale, and heralded as a dangerous threat at the other. Neither of these extremes is really fair. The Bristol Centre has a valuable therapeutic role to play in the management and control of cancer, and it has not set itself up with a view to seducing patients away from other helpful treatments.

Medicine has always been a glorious bundle of magic, method, psychology, science and common sense. For some reason doctors like to exaggerate the scientific component, but medicine has never been very scientific. It has its moments certainly, but just a glance at Archibald Cochrane's book *Effectiveness and Efficiency* will show that describing medicine as a science is wishful thinking on the part of those doctors who do. Why they should wish it to be a science is subject matter enough for another book. Perhaps they are afraid of their inadequacy when it comes to the loving, the understanding, the intuition, and the inspiration needed to operate outside the scientific model. The sight of a patient wired up to tens of thousands of pounds worth of equipment would be reassuring for a doctor, it would allow him to feel that everything possible is being done for that patient, and allow him to side-step the challenge of meeting the patient's tears and suffering on a personal level. Doctors must ask themselves whether, in these circumstances, the paraphernalia of high technology might act as a barrier to the development of a more personal relationship with their patients. If it does, then one must next ask: what has been lost? Is the possible alienation of patients in the short term justified by improvements in their condition in the long term? This is what we would all like to believe, but I am far from certain that it is always the case.

Unfortunately such is the dedication and devotion to this way of doing things, some practitioners continue to use these techniques, even when they have been shown *not* to work. This must mean that they have a preference for this way of treating people even when it may not be in the patient's interests. Dr Mather conducted an experiment in Bristol in 1971 to test the value of coronary care units (*BMJ*, vol 3, 1971). He found that intensive care was no more effective than just sending the patient home. He is not the first to suggest that patients are literally frightened to death by what has been described as an 'orgy of medical razzmatazz'. Perhaps even more interesting than his conclusion was the reaction of other cardiologists who showed an alarming unwillingness to have their methods evaluated. This is covered in detail in Professor Cochrane's book. The point of raising it here is to suggest that many who cry for proof do not heed it when it comes.

Insistence that all healing methods should be scientifically tested is a good way of keeping a lot of them at arm's length, since many holistic techniques cannot be tested in ways that are so popular with scientists. The double blind trial, for example, is possible with homoeopathy, but not with acupuncture.

In a talk he gave recently to the Oncology Club at Bristol Royal Infirmary, Professor Baum from King's College stated emphatically that while doctors are using such potentially dangerous treatments as chemotherapy and radiotherapy, the need to justify this with adequate proof lies heavily upon them. One could not possibly disagree with this, but there is a sense in which Bristol does not have the same need to justify itself because what we are doing is essentially safe and benign. Despite this we are currently engaged in two research programmes in keeping with the current passion for this type of assessment. But if a major objective of a therapeutic programme is that patients should feel better in themselves, then the only proof of this is how they actually feel, and the only test required to find out is to ask them. This kind of subjective data does not cut much ice with people educated to expect specific degrees of statistical significance, and I admit it raises difficulties for such people when it comes to accepting whether Bristol has anything useful to offer. It does not, however, raise any difficulties for the patients.

Despite the fact that doctors cling to the scientific aspect of medicine, the patient still holds an orientation that goes beyond this view. This will be expressed eloquently with remarks like 'Mr So-and-So is taking care of me', or 'I am in Professor Whatsit's hands.' This would suggest that patients are seeking a personal, indeed loving, relationship with their medicine man which may be at odds with his view of himself as a scientist. It may also be at odds with the way our medical services are structured as a result of the high-technology revolution. If much of doctors' work is to be done by drugs and machines – where verification is fairly easy – then that is where the money and resources will go. If doctors end up with two minutes allocated for face-to-face interaction that is hardly surprising. I don't think they can have it both ways: they cannot reasonably reach out for more and more complicated machinery and sophisticated drugs which have the effect of claiming the lion's share of resources and attention, and at the same time complain that there isn't enough time to talk to patients. The time that doctors spend with patients has to be paid for, and perhaps if they had the courage and confidence to fight for more time they would have less need of the machines.

I suspect that many doctors are most unhappy with the situation in which they find themselves, but feel helpless to change it. This may be reflected in the higher than usual levels of alcoholism and suicide amongst doctors. It is certainly true that a great many practitioners are genuinely frustrated in their wish to devote more time to discussion with their patients in order to establish a deeper awareness of why they are ill.

The argument that focusing all the attention on the physical body is so successful that it justifies any alienation of the patient's broader needs is a way of thinking that is not confined to conventional medicine. One of the most famous non-conventional metabolic therapies for cancer control, advocating the use of juices, coffee enemas, enzyme supplements and so on, has no place in it for a non-physical dimension. When I asked an official representative and proponent of these methods why they did not include stress control in the regime, the answer was that once the cancer was gone there would be no need for this, and anyway patients following their programme wouldn't have time. Sounds familiar doesn't it? This regime could not be called holistic any more than surgery could be called holistic. It may be radical and alternative in its methods, but it maintains the old paradigm of the doctor being in charge and the patient doing what he or she is told. Once the doctor invites the patient to become part of the healing process then the doctor relinquishes power. His expertise becomes only part of what is going on because the patient is supplying something of his own. Doctors are most certainly not the only therapists who have difficulty with this. I know plenty of acupuncturists who play the game of 'you just leave it all to me' and 'you wouldn't understand if I tried to explain'. There is a tendency to equate alternative medicine with holistic medicine and this is to miss the point. Alternative medicine is part of the whole in the same way that conventional medicine is part of the whole.

All therapists have devoted years of their lives to the search for knowledge and hours of effort and sacrifice in the perfection of their skills. They acquire a belief in, and a devotion to, their particular way of doing things and often promote it at the expense of anything else. Allowing a place for other approaches and techniques is sometimes very challenging and may be strongly resisted. Often the cry for scientific proof is nothing more than an excuse not to open up to new ideas that may not be accessible by the usual scientific routes.

The barrier that prevents therapists changing or adapting or expanding their way of doing things is not lack of evidence, it is the force of attachment. This is just as much of a trap for the acupuncturist or the herbalist as it is for the oncologist and cardiologist. When any therapist anywhere raises objections to patients seeking additional help and advice about his condition, then I think it is this attachment that we are up against. However, if doctors are genuinely distressed by the fact that the pressure under which they work leaves them very little time to minister to the patients' broader needs, then they will welcome the opportunity to send them to Bristol. Bristol is no threat to doctors who recognize the need for a wider medical model but find they cannot work within that model themselves. Only doctors who do not, at heart, believe in treating patients as a whole could see the Bristol Programme as a threat or an alternative.

THE PROGRAMME

At the moment we have the following therapeutic staff working at the Cancer Help Centre:

counsellors
trained teachers of relaxation, meditation, visualization, bio-feedback, breathing
nutritionists
art therapists
doctors and nurses
spiritual healers

When we first started the Centre we offered something that was then described as a 'metabolic therapy'. This included the use of substances like amygdalin and benzaldehyde and required the use of detoxification techniques like coffee enemas. We have modified and adapted this metabolic therapy considerably over the years and it is now much simpler. The regime is more manageable and our results are just as good.

One of the difficulties inherent in using amygdalin and benzaldehyde is that they *could* be dangerous and patients need a good deal of cooperation from their doctors when using such substances. This is not always forthcoming and our aim is to offer a regime that the patient can follow alone if necessary.

Our observations over the years have led us to believe that simplification and rationalization in the area of supplements has made life a lot easier for our patients with no apparent cost to progress.

We also believe that a patient can be helped as much, if not more, by learning to avoid being a high-cancer risk, rather than fighting off the manifestation of the disease. For this reason we have expanded and developed our psychological programme considerably. Almost daily various researches reveal more about the relationship between cancer and stress, and there is much talk about 'cancer personalities' and the importance of the right psychological attitude in recovery. Work in this area is now considered to be a most important aspect of our programme.

Our current educational and self-help programme offers our patients the opportunity to put together a lifestyle incorporating as many as possible of these aspects of healthy living:

stress control
good nutrition
vitamin and mineral supplements
positive visualization
oxygenating exercises
creativity
healing

We are well aware that although personality, diet, stress and some mineral deficiences have been linked to cancer as possible causative factors, there is little hard evidence to suggest that attending to such things when the disease is in evidence has a significant effect on it. The fact that something may be a predisposing factor does not automatically mean that reversing it will be therapeutic. But risk factors point us to areas that should be looked at closely and investigated fully. They are telling us something very important about the disease, and the more we understand about these factors the more we shall be able to construct something useful out of them in terms of its control. Perhaps working on combinations of risk factors will be the answer. Smoking may be an undisputed causative factor in relation to lung cancer, but just giving up cigarettes will not make it go away. Even so, who would not give such advice to a lung cancer patient? Working with risk factors in the way we do at Bristol has had some impressive results with our patients. In some patients changing the emotional, physical and spiritual environment seems to have the effect of starving the cancer of the nurturing it needs. It certainly does more than 'bolt the stable door'.

When we introduce new patients to our ideas we often show them this model. (Fig. 1). It demonstrates very simply the interaction between the different aspects of ourselves. We encourage them to see their hospital treatment in the framework of this model. It is important that we should understand that a truly holistic model will have a place in it for entirely physical treatments. One must respect and understand the fact that there are times when mechanistic, interventionist action must be taken, particularly if the life of the patient is in immediate danger. We also explain that some cancers respond well to medical treatment and, where there is a high success rate, we should welcome this. But it is still true a person's needs do not begin and end with the physical body, and patients are all too aware that hospitals tend to cater exclusively to their physical needs and that this is not enough.

Although the current trend in medical circles is towards a greater understanding of patients' broader needs, few hospitals have been able to make more than a token gesture in this direction. The Faith Courtauld unit at King's College Hospital and Professor Calman's work in Glasgow are impressive

A simple Holistic Model of Man
in relation to the Bristol Programme

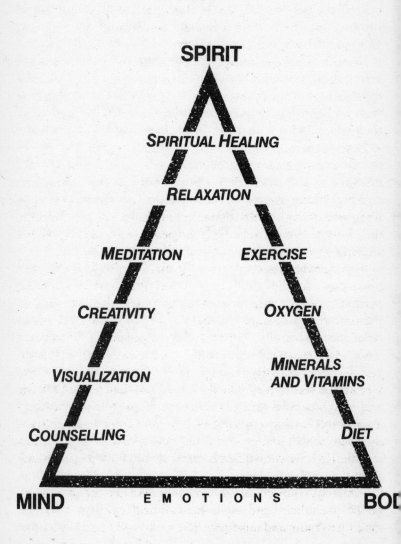

exceptions to this, and of course there are others, but by and large patients must look beyond the hospital if they wish to work with their emotional and spiritual needs. In fact, we encourage them to look beyond Bristol too, because we do not believe that any one institution or organization can possibly have all the answers. We see the Centre as a place where people can be educated both in a broader understanding of illness, and in wider ways of caring for themselves.

Nobody needs convincing that they have more than physical suffering to deal with. Patients can identify readily with, and have plenty to say about, mental and spiritual pain. Our first task at Bristol is to help them integrate these aspects of themselves and work on them simultaneously.

Despite the neat categories on the diagram, we should try not to compartmentalize everything. A holistic model is a dynamic model where everything is moving and interacting and everything affects everything else. The temptation is to wrap everything up in neat packets: diet and supplements for the physical body, counselling for peace of mind, healing for spiritual grace. In reality nothing works quite like that.

Anyone who has ever fasted for any length of time knows how, after a few days, they begin to feel quite wonderful. If you practise yoga or tai-chi or meditation at such a time it is particularly rewarding. Somehow it is easier to do, it seems to come more naturally. Although the recommended Bristol diet is not a fast, it can have the same cleansing and purifying effect, and this does actually make it easier to learn relaxation and meditation techniques. The Bible is full of examples of fasting and enlightenment going hand in hand, and this is a familiar association for Eastern mystics. So, although the diet affects the body, it will influence non-physical things as well. Studies in America have shown that diet affects behaviour, moods and feelings.

Similarly, counselling can have the effect of helping us to let go of prejudices and rigid behavioural patterns that are making us tense and miserable. We are bound to feel better for this mentally, but we are likely to feel better physically too. In a healthy way of doing things, we would discharge our emotions through sound and action, but most of us have been taught not to do this. Consequently we may suppress our emotions, holding them inside ourselves for years, undischarged and unexpressed. This creates considerable physical tension. Tension that we grow so used to having, we assume it to be normal. If we let go of these bottled-up feelings on a mental level, we will also experience great physical relief. Obviously this makes it easier for us to learn to relax, but it may improve our digestion, lead to more refreshing sleep and affect many other bodily actions.

Once we start to understand the interrelationship between every aspect of ourselves and our various therapies we will feel more inclined to move towards a truly holistic programme. We actively encourage patients to do this, not only with the methods we have to offer, but with treatments and therapies they pursue outside Bristol. If the medical model is big enough then it is easy to see a role for acupuncture, herbal medicine, surgery and prayer groups without conflict.

The problem for most patients is that they are deeply enmeshed with a materialist medical world that tends to concentrate exclusively on the physical body. It is hardly surprising that neither they nor their doctors can see a place for meditation, counselling or creativity in such a narrow model. Once we shift our perspective and take a wider view of disease and healing it is much easier to find a place for everything.

Naturally it is difficult to release ourselves from some of our long-held, deeply ingrained beliefs about illness. These might include the idea that once you have cancer, you can never get rid of it. Or that if you do have cancer you will not be able to lead a normal, active life. Even if we manage to replace these mind-sets with more positive and encouraging beliefs we are often stuck with friends and relatives who are thinking along the old lines. It is sad that the poor old patient, who already has plenty to cope with, should have to carry the burden of re-educating the world, but this is often the case.

For this, and other reasons, we encourage everyone who comes to Bristol to bring a friend or relative with them. This means that at least one person in the patient's orbit understands what he or she is trying to do. It also means that there is likely to be a bit more support and understanding when new and unusual foods start appearing on the table and time is taken away from the family or the office for relaxation and visualization. But, most importantly, it means that at least one other person in the patient's world is trying to break free of negative thinking and expand into a greater consciousness of health and healing.

One of the delightful bonuses for everyone associated with the Bristol programme is the effect these methods have on the accompanying relatives and friends. Week after week we hear about arthritic knees getting better, migraines dwindling to nothing, chronic backaches disappearing. This from the lips of people who are puzzled, but pleased, to find that paying some attention to the needs of the whole person – body, mind and spirit – can have some wonderfully unexpected outcomes.

Once we start looking thoughtfully into the holistic model we soon see that it is not about treatment or cures, it is about a wholesome, healthy way of living. A way of living that affords us the best possible potential for physical comfort and spiritual growth. This is practical and desirable for everyone, not just cancer patients. It is a way of being that the staff at Bristol are daily trying to put into action for themselves. It is the only sane way forwards for all of us.

Understandably, we will all have slightly different needs and therefore each one of us will adopt and adapt the various facets of this programme accordingly. We should be sensitive to what we need at any given time, not rigidly follow a prescribed pattern for the rest of our lives. There are days when we are in pain, when we may find healing and relaxation absorb our attention; other times when we are bubbling with creativity and can think of nothing else but going with the energy of that.

The danger lies in feeding one part of ourselves at the

expense of another. Years of authoritarian schooling and parenting have usually left us quite comfortable with the work ethic. Most people are very good at tackling and achieving difficult tasks. People like this may go at the diet aspect of the programme like a bull at a gate, and report back to Bristol that they have been 'good' and not 'failed'. (Recognize the vocabulary of the old school report?) But they may find it difficult to do something they enjoy, just for the sake of doing it, something creative. It would be hard for them not to think this would be 'lazy' or 'indulgent' or just a waste of time.

Because it may be hard for us to know what our personal bias might be, we encourage patients to try to explore as many facets of themselves and these therapies as they can. In this way they will gradually come to know the difference between prejudice and intuition.

2

Nutrition and Physical Therapies

'Your food should be your medicine: your medicine your food.' *Hippocrates*
'The major cancers of our time are diet-caused, mainly by fat and cholesterol.' *Dr Ernst Wynder addressing US Senate Select Committee on Nutrition and Human Needs*

DIET

The first part of the Bristol Programme that visitors to the Cancer Help Centre will experience is the diet.

Nothing excites more debate or controversy than the role of nutrition in the control of cancer. Otherwise perfectly mature and sensible people have been known to lose their reason completely when faced with someone who thinks 'they are what they eat'. Any vegetarian will tell you that the simple act of refusing animal protein can sometimes elicit responses verging on physical violence from a few dedicated carnivores. I think the reason for this has something to do with the fact that there is an implied criticism floating around, mixed up with a few moral prescriptives about what is 'right' or 'wrong'. This has the effect of putting people on the defensive, and, as we all know, one popular form of defence is attack – hence the occasional heavy reactions to the health-food freaks. If this can happen amongst ordinary mortals with no medical axe to grind you will not be surprised to hear that doctors are often very sensitive to the food-and-health debate. After all, if it does matter what you eat, then why didn't they tell you that, instead of leaving you to find it out for yourself?

The reason is likely to be simple: the doctor probably doesn't know anything about nutrition. Despite the fact the Hippocrates is reverentially acknowledged as 'the father of modern medicine' his ideas about nutrition went out just as fast as advanced technological food production came in. Because there was *enough* to eat we were fooled into thinking it didn't matter *what* we ate. Now we know better, of course, and every supermarket on a Saturday sees crowds of anxious wives trying to juggle with calculating the polyunsaturates and the monosaturates and taking the answer away from the required level of Essential Fatty Acids, in order to lower cholesterol levels in their obese husbands who are outside smoking themselves to death in the car. Now that we know we may be digging our graves with our teeth we are often more frightened and guilty, but very often none the wiser.

At one time or another I have read so many books that have either implied or directly stated that cancer can be brought about by faulty diet that I wish to make one thing clear right away: although I have met people for whom I believe that faulty nutrition might have been instrumental in their development of cancer, I have met far more for whom I do not believe this to be true. It can be most annoying to be told that your poor eating habits have led to the development of a life-threatening disease. Particularly if you happen to have been sharing a table with someone whose eating habits are the same, if not worse, than yours, and there appears to be nothing at all the matter with them. Very trying. Not half as annoying as being something of a health-food-macrobiotic-organic-nut and vegetarian to boot, and still developing a tumour. That was me. Let's be clear about this: diet may or may not be relevant as a causative factor, but I think it is definitely worth looking at in terms of therapy.

When I first set out to use diet as part of a cancer fighting programme I was appalled by the amount of disagreement there seemed to be. I used to sit sore-eyed, night after night, ploughing my way through an apparently endless supply of books that all seemed to be annoyingly contradictory in one way or another. Naturally they all claimed to be the final and ultimate word of truth. I know from talking to patients at Bristol that this is an experience shared by many. As a result, some people give up on the idea of dietary changes altogether, but this would be a mistake. We must not throw the baby out with the bath water. There may be large areas of dispute about how to use diet as a therapy, but there are large areas of agreement as well. Let's look at those.

After agonizing for several weeks about whether or not it was safe to eat oranges (yes, even something as apparently innocent as an orange has its detractors as well as its devotees), I decided to make a list of all the things that everyone agreed about and start there. This left me with a manageable set of dietary rules which line up very well with the basic nutritional guidelines that we use at Bristol.

1. Reduce protein intake in general and animal protein in particular.
2. Reduce levels of fat.
3. Eat as much natural food as possible.
4. Eat as much raw food as possible.
5. Avoid salt.
6. Avoid sugar.
7. Avoid stimulants.
8. Think positively about what you are eating.

Let's look at these in a bit more detail.

First, the protein issue

At one time it was believed that the enzymes required to digest proteins in food were being diverted from their more important role of breaking down the polypeptide coating with which cancer cells protect themselves from destruction by the immune system. Bradford, a great pioneer of the use of laetrile in cancer control, held this view, but I have not been able to find any evidence other than his to support it. However, it may be true. What we do have is evidence to suggest that groups of people who gather protein from non-animal sources (and are therefore likely to be eating less protein than the average carnivore) have much lower levels of cancer than is common in other population groups. The Mormons, for example, and the Seventh Day Adventists, share satisfyingly low cancer statistics (H. Seidman, *Environmental Research*, vol 3, 1970). Of course this may be due to other factors, not just the meat-eating. It may just be really nice to be a Mormon. There are other things about these groups that they have in common other than their attitude to animal protein, but vegetarian groups seem to exhibit this low cancer tendency and we should take account of this when thinking about the best diet to prevent or control cancer.

Unfortunately most of us are pretty unimaginative about alternative sources of protein and fly from the lamb chops to the cheese. This is not a good idea because dairy products are not in our interests right now. The dietician and kitchen staff at Bristol advise about the use of pulses, peas, beans, wholegrain rice, wholewheat bread and so on as protein-rich meat substitutes. Don't be alarmed by accusations that some of these may be 'second-class proteins'. This remark is based on the fact that some protein sources contain the full string of amino acids that make up the protein chain, whereas non-animal sources contain only a few of these amino acids. The way round this problem is to eat several protein-rich foods at the same time, and this is exactly what you will do if you are consciously feeding yourself a varied, wholefood diet.

Dr Alfred Harper (Food and Nutrition Board of the National Research Council, USA) says, 'Some proteins provide more limited amounts of some amino-acids than others. But it has been recognized that if you increase the quantity you don't have to worry about the quality. We have shown that adults can remain in protein balance on a diet of wheat, even flour.'

The question as to how much protein we need is very difficult to answer. Some of the early nutritional regimes pioneered for cancer patients advocated very low protein intake because these therapists were strongly influenced by the idea that the enzymes needed to digest the protein in the diet would be put to better use digesting the protective coating of the cancer cells. One such therapist (William Kelly) meted out marginal amounts of protein by allowing only a tiny handful of almonds a day. . . . But we must set this against other suggestions (Issels') that we need one gram of protein per kilogram of body weight daily. I think the uncertainty and anxiety we generate when we start struggling with details at this level leads to us losing more than we gain. There *is* some evidence that a vegetarian diet is in our interest, but to date there is no evidence that eating nine almonds a day is better than tucking into lentil soup with wholewheat rolls followed by a baked potato or whatever. However, the amount of protein needed will vary according to the extent of the cancer in the body. Tumours can become very protein-greedy and they will feed themselves at the expense of the rest of the body. If you think this might apply to you then keep your protein levels up and get advice. You may actually need protein powder as a supplement.

A key aspect of the protein issue involves the source and quality of protein rather than the quantity. Animal husbandry leaves a lot to be desired. We are all perfectly well aware of this although our reactions are different. Some of us get terribly worked up about it, join groups and protest for animal rights. Others among us sigh wearily and accept what is going on because we feel there is nothing we can do to stop it. None of us, I think, could reasonably deny that the interests of the manufacturer usually take precedence over the interests of the animal. What is much more frightening is that the interests of the manufacturer often take precedence over the interests of the consumer. It is not good for *us* to have meat and poultry fattened by the addition of hormone supplements in their food: this is good for sales and good for profits. We cannot afford to be naïve about this. There is considerable evidence that links certain cancers to hormone activity. Women with cancer of the breast, ovaries or uterus and men with cancer of the testes or prostate are almost routinely treated with hormone therapy. This is because some tumours contain receptors which take up and feed on particular hormones. If we can reduce the levels of these hormones in the blood then, theoretically, we can help to 'starve' the tumour. Thousands of women with cancer are given a drug designed to reduce their oestrogen levels, many of them will even have their ovaries removed to this end. It is nothing short of madness to spend half one's life trying to reduce oestrogen levels with such dramatic and invasive techniques, and the other half tucking into chicken wings that have been plumped to perfection by the judicious use of just such hormones.

As I write this I have a mental picture of Mr-Bullock-From-The-Meat-Marketing-Syndicate coming at me from behind with a meat cleaver in one hand and lots of documents full of information about 'permitted' and 'safe' levels in the other. It does not comfort me to hear that substances are used in the rearing and preparation of livestock that at some point would *not* be permitted and would be *un*safe. I think it is best not to take the risk.

Being thoughtfully aware of these factors means that if later we chose to return to a meat-eating diet we can at least make an effort to find animals reared by farmers who don't go in for these methods. And if you are thinking this will be difficult and expensive, well, yes it might be to begin with, but times are changing fast and they will change even faster if the consumer demands it. When I was first ill the only way to get organic vegetables was to grow your own. Now there is an ever-growing list of suppliers, and even supermarket chains are responding to the demand. No doubt the same will be true for meat from safely reared animals.

Some people are devoted, natural carnivores: my husband for one. 'If God had meant us to be vegetarian He wouldn't have invented Tournedos Rossini' – you know the type. If reintroducing meat to your diet is one of your long-term goals then be prepared to lobby for something safe to eat. In the meantime, look for non-animal protein sources, it's safer.

The significance of fat

Evidence suggests that fat may be implicated in the development of cancer. Since we have come to accept that it already plays a role in cardiovascular disorders we may not find this too hard to believe. Unfortunately the torrent of publicity surrounding the desperate struggle for the commercial market has led to a great deal of cynicism. Battles take place nightly between TV mothers in tracksuits, unpacking low-cholesterol family picnics in daisy-strewn fields, and their seductive counterparts who lounge around in their négligées, breakfasting in chrome-glittering sunlounges, festooned with houseplants, smiling indulgently at their husbands who have just discovered to their surprise that they are Back to Butter. As if this wasn't bad enough, we are now faced with a new range of competitors in the guise of low-fat spreads. These look, and often taste, like something for oiling the sewing machine. If the E-numbers are anything to go by, they probably have about the same nutritional value, but the big selling point is that they don't make you fat.

I do admit that against this kind of cultural chaos it is difficult to simplify the fat issue, but we must try. The good news is that the move towards a vegetarian diet will dramatically reduce the levels of fat in our diet. The not-so-good news is that we cannot substitute for meat all the usual favourites like eggs, milk and cheese which are high in protein, because they are also high in fat. Hence the Bristol preference for beans and pulses and whole grains.

Just when we think we are getting the hang of this someone will tell us that fat is an absolutely essential part of our diet and without certain basic levels we shall not be able to function at all. True. But some fats are more useful than others, some more potentially hazardous. One of the reasons why meat may be implicated in the cancer scene is because it is so high in fat and the hormones in it are fat soluble. But there is no need to make this more complicated than necessary: fats that coagulate, set stickily on your plate, or go hard when cold are the ones to avoid. Out with the dripping from the Sunday roast and in with the sunflower oil. Using 'soft' instead of 'hard' fats means you are moving away from saturated to unsaturated fats, which is in your interests from just about every health angle you care to look.

The most healthy of all fats are those found in certain fish oils, and later when you are concentrating on maintaining good health rather than acquiring it, you may be advised to include some fish in your diet. That is if you aren't a convert to vegetarianism by then.

As with anything, it is possible to start nit-picking over the relative value of safflower oil as compared with sunflower oil, and then get lost in a maze of detail that probably won't affect our progress much one way or another. Remember to let simplicity win the day if anxiety is the alternative.

Eat as much natural food as possible

You can cut a wide swathe through all the discussions surrounding what constitutes a 'natural' food by just asking yourself what has happened to what you are eating since it left its source. If it started out as a seed:

has it been fertilized?
has it been dried?

has it been frozen?
has it been preserved?
has it been coloured?
has it been flavoured?
was it picked raw and left to ripen on board ship?
has it been sprayed to stop it ripening too soon?
has it been stir-fried, boiled, marinated or stewed?

The list of possible questions is endless. It certainly isn't necessary to ask or answer very many to get an idea of what I mean. What you eat should be as near to its natural, growing state as you can reasonably find it. This means goodbye to all those instant meals – of the 'just add water and stir' variety – all the handy packages and tins, in fact just about everything that lines the supermarket shelves.

There are basically two reasons for this apparently heartless ban. Let's take the question of additives first: the list of unpronounceable, unintelligible extras which the manufacturers soothingly assure us are all 'permitted'. Many of the dyes, preservatives, emulsifiers and sweeteners in regular current use have a doubtful record and are often extremely harmful if used in anything other than the 'permitted' amounts. And how can we be sure that, even if the tinned chicken chunks genuinely do contain only the appropriately safe level of preservative, by serving it with the latest packet sauce mix we are not raising this to an unacceptably high dose? The people who make the tinned chicken chunks can be reasonably sure that you won't eat more than a tin a day, but they can't possibly know what else you are eating. Who knows what deadly cocktails we are mixing up for ourselves when we feed ourselves this kind of food. How much of this toxic rubbish might we accumulate over the years? How can we sensibly talk of 'permitted' levels?

I am not too frightened of being drowned in a vat of carrot juice by managing directors of big food companies because I could build myself a substantial liferaft from the quantities of books written on the subject of E-numbers which are attracting so much attention . . .

The second reason for avoiding processed food is that it is dead. It has also lost many vitamins and minerals that are very valuable to you right now.

Eat as much raw food as possible

At Bristol we encourage patients to eat a high percentage of their food raw. By doing this we feel that the maximum nutritional value is gained because none of the vitamins and minerals have been leached out in the cooking process. But this also means that more of the food eaten is 'living' and it may be that living food really does have a quality about it that is important. I say 'may' because we are firmly and squarely in the area of supposition now: as far as I know nobody has been able to prove this in any scientific sense although the anecdotal evidence is considerable and many people feel passionately that vital, living food is regenerative in a very special way. Leslie Kenton's book (see page 61) is positively inspirational on this subject.

Although we encourage patients who come to Bristol to eat as much raw food as they possibly can, we know that this will vary a great deal from person to person. There are always a few dedicated enthusiasts who eat 70 or even 80 per cent of their daily diet in a raw, uncooked state. Other patients view these individuals with a combination of admiration and despair because for them this would be impossible or impractical. Much depends on how well we can chew and break up uncooked food: this is a lot easier if we have good, strong teeth, and full use of our gastro-intestinal tract. Many patients are having to manage without either of these advantages and may be suffering from cancer in the mouth, throat, stomach or bowel, and for them it might be very difficult to eat large amounts of raw food. Adapt the question of raw food to your own capacity. Don't eat more than feels comfortable.

If raw, organically grown food is the nearest we get to its

natural state, then raw food that is still growing will definitely get you extra Brownie points. It is not actually necessary for you to kneel in the allotment and start munching in order to achieve this degree of sophistication. This nutritional programme can be tough on your social life, I admit, but you can still eat with the family. The best single source of raw, living food is sprouted grains. If your immediate reaction to this is that it's all too complicated, think again. The chances are that you have already done quite a bit of sprouting. In fact I would go so far as to say that anyone who has spent enough time in the school system to learn to read this book will not have been able to avoid growing mustard and cress on the windowsill. Most beans and seeds will sprout given enough time, moisture and warmth. Some things – like alfafa and wheatgrass – are almost legendary in the cancer-control stories, so this is something well worth the effort.

Don't worry: you won't turn into a beaded, ear-ringed commune leader overnight, in fact such an expert won't come within a mile of you if you don't make a better job of sprouting grains than I did. Not wishing to be negative and dwell on my own failures (that's another book) I confess to creating a lot of slimy, smelly messes which gave the compost a terrific boost, but did nothing for my morale, never mind my cancer. Finally my husband tracked down a splendid little item consisting of a series of stacked plastic trays, with which even I manage to succeed. Most health food shops stock these or will know where to get you one. They will also be full of good advice on how to manage with blotting paper, jam jars etc., and I wish you all the best.

Mung beans are noted for their capacity to germinate quickly in almost any conditions but are also renowned for their potentially disastrous effect on any weak teeth or bridgework. This is occasioned by the crafty way some of them lie doggo amongst their soft, chewy brothers, revealing themselves in the mouth with shocking abruptness and the consistency of a small pebble. Apart from this there do not appear to be many hazards associated with sprouting grains, which is fortunate since you are heartily recommended to get to grips with this and make it a regular part of your diet.

Avoid salt

Nothing new about this, in fact you are probably sick of hearing it. Salt has been having a consistently bad press lately in view of its undisputed connection with the rise of cardio-vascular disease. Many people have already made some effort to cut down on salt intake but for those of you intrepid and defiant enough to have ignored all the warnings, I am afraid the advice for cancer patients is what you might expect. No salt.

In reality you will be getting some salt, but at Bristol we suggest you avoid using it in cooking or adding it at the table. Many of the foods we eat contain salt naturally, so you will be taking some even if you are making a conscious effort to avoid it. This is just as well since a certain amount of sodium – and it is sodium we're talking about – is essential for the body's needs. These needs will be met by the presence of sodium in the food you are eating, so forget all those dramas about Great Uncle Alfred being saved in the nick of time by being force-fed on salt tablets: he was in the tropics, marching about with the mad dogs in the noonday sun and sweating out his precious supplies. Nothing like that is happening to you.

There was a time when man was not able to find salt regularly or in any great quantities and some early civilizations regarded salt as a priceless commodity. As if in sympathy with this the body stores sodium well and, although it is lost through diarrhoea and excessive perspiration, the kidneys are programmed to keep salt levels in the urine at around 2 per cent. This is why you must not drink the sea water while floating parched and dehydrated on your raft. Sea water is at least 3 per cent salt, often much more, and your kidneys will steal fluid from other tissues rather than pass out saltier urine. You don't need a degree in biochemistry to see now why you should hang on until the Air Sea Rescue crowd arrive. Or to see why sodium levels in the body can become unacceptably high.

There is a sensitive relationship between sodium and potassium in the body and an excess of sodium has the effect of reducing potassium levels. As excess sodium enters the cells (in the body's effort to maintain extra-cellular sodium levels within fine limits) potassium levels in the cells fall. This leads to fluid retention and the potential for increased blood pressure. Not only this, many nutritionists believe that cancer is associated with low levels of potassium and advise a diet rich in potassium. Obviously this requires that sodium levels should be kept down. Many experts in the control of cancer through nutrition hold this view and some even give high supplements of potassium, at least in the early stages of therapy. Gerson went so far as to say 'the beginning of all chronic disease in the body is due to loss of potassium from the cells'.

By adopting a diet high in raw and natural food you will automatically be reducing your salt intake. Dried, tinned, packaged and processed food contains an enormous amount of added salt. It may surprise you to read the listed contents of packaged food and see how high up you find the salt. There's a lot of 'hidden' salt around for the unwary.

Ross Horne, in his book *The New Health Revolution*, describes salt as 'a harmful irritant conducive to high blood pressure, cardiovascular disease, kidney damage, oedema, arthritis, migraine and cancer'. He also refers to the fact that the high incidence of stomach cancer in Japan is thought to be related to a high salt diet. If after all this you still find it difficult to adjust your taste you could try using Ruthmol – a high potassium salt substitute – to flavour your food. But in the long term it is better to try to wean yourself off the habit of seeking a salty taste in what you eat. Substitutes keep the addiction alive and prevent the development of a more subtle palate in the appreciation of food.

Avoid sugar

People have filled whole books with detailed descriptions of the danger associated with high sugar consumption. Unfortunately we don't seem to be taking much notice since average consumption is rising at a terrifying rate.

Ross Horne says, 'All refined carbohydrates, including raw sugar, treacle, molasses and processed honey, whether in drinks, cakes, confectionery or other forms, can cause disruption to normal blood chemistry with adverse physical and mental effects; such as hypoglycemia, headaches, depression, hyperactivity, irrational or violent behaviour, high blood viscosity, angina etc.' (I like that little 'etc.' don't you: there's not much left after that!)

Sugar is, quite simply, bad for you. There is no place for sugar in a nutritional programme designed to maximize health and performance.

Even if you don't have the proverbial Sweet Tooth you may be eating more than you ever thought possible. Ross Horne tells us, for example, that tomato ketchup contains more sugar than some icecreams; that powdered cream substitute for coffee contains more sugar than the famous Hershey bars; that some of the most popular breakfast cereals contain over 50 per cent sugar? Did you know that? Probably not.

Apart from the health risks associated with it, one of the most dangerous things about sugar is that it provides calories without nutrition. In other words you get energy but no food value. This means that you will lose your appetite for other food that does have nutritional value, food that can actually help you in the fight against cancer. Even worse, this empty substance, itself devoid of vitamins, requires vitamin B1 in the process of being metabolized by the body. In order to digest sugar, which is no use to use at all, we have to part with some of our stores of vitamin B, which is very serious indeed. It is likely that chronically low levels of vitamin B1, for example, cause underactivity of the thyroid which in turn may lead to high cholesterol levels and all the health problems associated with that. Low levels of vitamin B in general will affect the myelination of nerves, and high sugar intake is often associated with nervous tissue degeneration.

Honey is a derivative of plant nectar and is high in the sugars fructose and glucose. However, if it has not been tampered with in any way, it may still contain some nutrients, mineral salts and enzymes and therefore qualify as a food. However it should be used sparingly. As with salt it is better to train yourself to accept new tastes in food than try to replicate old ones.

Sugar causes stress in the digestive system and the body has to work hard to keep it at acceptable levels in the blood. The pancreas and the liver are constantly struggling to produce insulin and glycogen just to keep a stable level. This uses up a lot of energy, vitamins and minerals that could be put to better use. Sugar does you no good whatsoever and has been shown time and again to be an agent of disease. Avoid it.

Avoid stimulants

I expect that by now you're thinking you could do with a few stimulants, but think again. The most prevalent and popular stimulant is caffeine which has long been considered a contributory cause of cancer and heart disease. Caffeine and tannin have the effect of blocking prostaglandin synthesis. This is a key component in all body functions and should be stimulated rather than inhibited.

Not only coffee but also tea, cocoa and cola contain caffeine. Caffeine is a highly stimulating, addictive substance and it is sometimes very difficult to give up. The harder it is the more you need to do it. It causes artificial stimulation of the nervous system and results in numerous effects similar to those of adrenalin. It dilates blood vessels and stimulates the heart which may beat arhythmically and erratically. The formation in the stomach of nitrosamines, some of which are carcinogens, is increased tenfold when even small amounts of coffee are consumed.

Unfortunately the many cups of tea and coffee we take during the course of a day have become enmeshed with our social life and this makes the habit difficult to break from the behavioural point of view as well. Of course there are lots of so-called substitutes on the market, but anyone who settles down to one of these in the innocent belief that it will bear anything but a verbal relationship to the real thing is in for a very disappointing evening. This is the difficulty with all substitutes: they delay the re-educating process and cause high levels of frustration. As long as we are not expecting drinks like chamomile or Bambu to taste like tea and coffee than we stand a chance of adapting to the new tastes. I have developed a great liking for dandelion coffee but that may be partly because my teenage children insist on calling Barleycup 'Barleycrap' and a mother can take just so much . . .

Be cautious with the use of spices in cooking. Some people feel they are irritants and that some may even be carcinogenic. I don't think we should over-react to this but it would be better to concentrate on herbs for flavouring whenever possible.

Strictly speaking alcohol is not a stimulant at all, in fact it depresses the function of all living cells. We are under the illusion that it stimulates us because, as it lessens the activity of the brain, it deadens anxiety. It affects judgement, concentration and self-control and may therefore render shy people quite chatty, nervous people more confident. This may make the party go with a swing but at a fairly high price. Alcohol is fermented sugar; it is consumed at the expense of vitamin B6 and it is hard work for the liver where the detoxification takes place. Cancer patients are already overworking their livers in the process of detoxifying the by-products of cancer cells and some of the drugs used in treatment. We need to be kind to the liver, not load it up with more work.

Even so, alcohol has been the subject of heated debate. Although on the face of it, it does sound terribly bad for you it is still true that several surveys have shown that people who drink small amounts often live longer and suffer fewer illnesses than people who don't drink at all. This is hard to reconcile with what we know about the effects of alcohol unless the stress-reducing, pleasure element is more significant than we imagined. One scientific study that did put in a good word for it suggested that a combination of oil of the evening primrose (linoleic acid), vitamin C and small amounts of alcohol, together produced a healthy boost to the immune system. On this basis I was advised by Josef Issels to allow myself a glass or two of wine and this is one aspect of my personal experience that has been carried on into the Bristol regime. Our doctors and nutritionists are prepared to see you weaving the occasional drink into your daily plan, although some patients prefer not to have any at all.

Think positively about what you are eating

Years ago I watched a sprightly looking man of 106 being interviewed by a keen television reporter who wanted to know what he had been eating all these years to account for his exceptional longevity and evident good health. 'I don't think it matters much what you eat,' he said, 'I think it matters what you think while you're eating it.'

When I was very ill I was sometimes inspired and comforted by the thought that every time I sat down to a well-balanced meal I was giving myself a therapeutic remedy, but there were times when I groaned inwardly at what I saw as another pile of rabbit food. We are all accustomed to awarding ourselves certain foods as a treat or a reward or a comfort and it is hard not to continue with these expectations even when the food we are eating is not what we would choose to reward or comfort ourselves with. At these times we may feel disappointed and frustrated by our new diet and we should not be too hard on ourselves when this happens. We need to balance the nutritional and physical gains against any emotional losses that come through feelings of anxiety and irritation. Allowing for an initial period of readjustment while you change your eating habits you should finally end up with a therapeutic diet that you enjoy. This is sometimes a difficult balance to achieve. Either we are ferociously hard on ourselves, never allowing any treats, letting the diet become a penance, or we are too sloppy and undisciplined and fail to benefit from the healing potential of good nutrition.

As well as using food as a comfort and a reward, many people use it subconsciously as a sedative. This may mean that a diet like the one suggested here may make them feel uncomfortable and more aware of emotional pain for a while, because they are missing the deadening effect of rich food. This is an effect that will pass given time.

I headed this chapter with an unequivocal quotation from a man who believes that diet is a key causative factor in relation to cancer. This is an opinion shared by many others, but at Bristol we do not hold such a hard and fast view. We have seen cases where it seemed as if faulty eating habits had been the last straw, the final insult that led to the slow deterioration of the body's capacity to stay well, but we have also seen cancers that we felt had little, if anything, to do with diet. This means that we try to adapt our advice about food and eating habits to accord with the needs of each individual. As a result we have ended up with an attitude towards nutrition that evokes a wide range of criticism.

I have been rather amused over the years to hear Bristol being criticized by doctors for being too strict about diet and by naturopaths for not being strict enough. It is certainly true that some people have come to us, had a go at the regime, set themselves impossibly high standards which they simply couldn't keep, felt guilty and ashamed, didn't dare to come back, ended up depressed, anxious and telling their doctors they felt worse than ever. We do everything it is humanly possible to do at Bristol in order to prevent this happening. We do not insist on a rigid, inflexible set of dietary rules. The problem is that most cancer patients are already frightened and a little bit fixated. It is very difficult for someone who feels under the threat of death not to become anxious, maybe even neurotic. I should know, I was as anxious and neurotic as it was possible to be. I tore into the whole idea of diet as therapy in the most rigid and self-punishing way imaginable. Nobody was forcing me to do this, I was forcing it on myself. My colleagues and I have seen many patients do this to themselves despite our protestations that they should not be so fierce or set such impossibly difficult goals. The guilt and shame that some patients express to their doctors is coming from them, not from pressure applied by therapists at Bristol. Indeed part of the programme at Bristol is to help patients understand more about this tendency to programme ourselves to fail, to alert them to the wiles of the 'internal saboteur'.

On the other hand we face criticism from naturopaths and other natural therapists for being too lenient and easy-going. It is certainly true that, by comparison with some of the nutritional schemes for cancer that I have studied over the years, the Bristol diet is a veritable picnic. If patients are temperamentally suited to a stricter regime, then we are happy to oblige, but the perfect therapeutic diet is what feels right and acceptable to each individual. If your diet is making you feel moody and miserable then you haven't got it right.

People often ask, 'Does it matter that I can't get organically grown food?' Of course, if there is a straightforward and simple choice, then organically grown food is better. Much better. But often the choice is far from simple and straight-forward. Some people live in the country and have access to their own or other peoples' allotments and enjoy the services of local shops that stock fresh produce from organic farms, but they are the lucky ones. For city dwellers the search for organically grown food may involve hours of time and a great deal of money. The additional effort and the financial burden of this may become so stressful that it is quite simply not worth it. All of us, however keen and strict we are, end up sometimes having to shop at the local supermarket. Some people have to compromise and do that most of the time. The trick is to be as selective as possible, prepare the food with love and eat it with a prayer. One day the world will come to its senses and we shall only be able to buy organically grown food. In the meantime we may have to compromise.

Whenever there are decisions to be made we must check and see whether anxiety figures in the calculation. We might put ourselves on the most wonderful diet in the world, but undo much of the good it does us because we never stop worrying about it, agonizing over every detail and wearing ourselves out in the process. For this reason alone we should never compare ourselves with what other people are doing. Obviously these nutritional rules are going to be easier for some to follow than others. The challenge is far greater if we have kitchen cupboards bursting with tins and instant microwave meals and a touchy bunch of teenagers super-sensitive to the slightest hint of change. In these circumstances I don't advise doing everything at once by having a clean sweep at home and denuding the local health-food store. Give yourself time to acquire new cooking skills, work your way in gently. Then you won't be weeping with despair because all the brown rice burnt to the pan and the rest of the family went out for chips. Setting too high a standard in the beginning invites a sense of failure and makes you more inclined to give up. This is true of all the new techniques described in this book.

With regard to the diet, I suggest you take it a meal at a time. First of all get yourself organized over breakfast, experiment with that for a while. Then move on to the midday and evening meals. There will always be people who make dramatic overnight changes, just like there are people who give up smoking instantly, but some of us need more time and patience. Be kind and sensitive to yourself. I often cheer up the Bristol patients by regaling them with tales of patients who misheard or misunderstood something, sailed away, did it all wrong and still came back looking and feeling marvellous. My favourite lady (not actually one of our patients) failed to grasp that she was allowed a *slice* of bread a day and proceeded to eat a *loaf* of bread a day. None the worse for this she recovered so completely she has become a legend in her own time.

Try to apply these eating guidelines with a bit of common sense. There is all the difference in the world between using one egg to bind a dozen nut rissoles, and frying up two for breakfast. If in doubt about anything, ask yourself these two questions: Is this doing me any good? and, Is this doing me any harm? More than likely there will be things that are not doing you any harm even if they aren't doing you much good. Provided they are giving you pleasure and enjoyment it won't hurt you too much to go ahead.

Suggested reading
The Bristol Recipe Book by Sadhya Rippon (Century Hutchinson) is the best recipe book for people wanting to follow the Bristol Programme.
Raw Energy by Lesley Kenton (Century Hutchinson).
The Holistic Cook by Janet Hunt (Thorsons) has a lot of useful information, but you have to pick and choose because she uses dairy products and meat in some of her recipes.
Taste of Life by Julie Stafford (Souvenir Press), is very good. Written by a woman who was cooking to save her husband's life. Also some meat and dairy products, but excellent in general.
The Cranks Recipe Book (J. M. Dent) is a classic. Written for vegetarians but fairly free with dairy products.

SUPPLEMENTS

As soon as possible after their arrival at the Centre patients will be seen individually by a doctor. Among other things they will discuss the most suitable vitamin and mineral schedule for that particular person.

A question I am often asked is why it should be necessary to supplement one's diet at all – least of all the diet recommended here. There is a strong school of thought that believes the whole vitamin and mineral business is excess to requirements and that anyone eating a balanced diet will get all the nutrients they need. This is an encouraging and appealing thought, but I don't think we can depend on it being the case. Methods of food production and preparation have changed over the years with deleterious effects on nutrients. It is often said that the populations of industrial societies are overfed and under-nourished. Even if it were true that a healthy person eating a high-quality diet could take in all the vitamins and minerals required to stay well, it is almost certainly true that extra nutrients are required to cope with stress or disease. In the case of the cancer patient it is likely that there are chronic deficiencies, ones that have been developing slowly for years, which need to be rectified. Such a person would soak up considerable quantities of supplements before reaching acceptable levels. Only after this point has been reached would it make sense to see vitamins and minerals as a treatment. Of course whether one can ever see supplements as potential healing therapy is the subject of fairly heated debate anyway.

Less contentious is the idea that extra vitamins and minerals may help reduce the side effects of cancer treatments. Radio-therapy, chemotherapy and, perhaps to a lesser extent, surgery destroy a wide range of vitamins in the body, but I have never heard of patients being given a routine course of supplements as part of their hospital treatment, although most people would agree this would be prudent.

The vitamin and mineral business is a vast subject covered at great length and in great detail in books devoted to this topic alone. Perhaps for this reason, a simple introduction to the whys and wherefores of the use of supplements will be an acceptable alternative to getting caught up in highly technical debates. Even so, the first thing that must be said is that each individual's needs will be different, and these remarks must be taken as the broad generalities they are. In order to make information in this book as accessible as possible I have tried to follow up theory with practice so that the reader can start to put a programme of some sort into action straight away. In keeping with this I have included advice about levels of self-medication that our doctors feel would be safe and acceptable. However, if you want to get the maximum benefit from a vitamin and mineral schedule, it would be best to have a personal blood analysis done.

This requires a brief visit to a doctor who will take a small blood sample from your arm which is sent off for detailed analysis. I say 'detailed' because the kind of analysis needed is not done as a matter of routine and it will be necessary for your doctor to be clear and specific in his request to the pathology laboratory about what he wants them to do. Since this is sometimes new to both doctor and patient alike, it may be quicker and simpler to send the sample away for analysis on the continent. There are several laboratories that specialize in this service. They will supply on request the equipment necessary to post and pack the blood sample, and give you their recommendations about what to take, and in what doses, on the basis of their findings. This kind of professional advice is invaluable because there is a synergistic effect at work with vitamins and minerals which makes therapy of this kind much more sophisticated than it might at first appear.

Nature's Own will supply names and addresses of organizations that offer this service, and arrange it for you. Or you may find that your local naturopath has a connection with someone who does it. It would be worth asking around. There are many different ways of establishing vitamin and mineral levels. Some practitioners use hair analysis instead of blood. If you make enquiries you may hear someone local to you being highly recommended. Equally you may find that your doctor is cooperative and helpful and you need look no further than your surgery.

One way or another, it should be possible to get a full and detailed analysis of your requirements, but if you want to get going straight away and work out the refinements later, here is the schedule we often give our patients at Bristol.

Vitamin C

A water soluble anti-oxidant essential for many body processes. It is interesting that man shares with the guinea pig a characteristic that sets us apart from all other primates: we cannot manufacture or store this vitamin in the body. We have to rely on outside sources and we have to take in regular supplies.

Uses Helps to metabolize fats, carbohydrates and amino acids. Protects tissues, especially cell membranes, against oxidative damage by chemically active 'free radicals'. Neutralizes sodium nitrate and sodium nitrite which are potent carcinogens. It has an important oxygen-carrying function.

Dose The minimum protective dose of ascorbic acid against clinical scurvy is 10 mg daily, but this does not provide a satisfactory vitamin allowance, which for adults ranges between 30–60 mg daily. Individuals vary greatly in their requirements and the higher the metabolic rate, the greater the requirement. Having just enough of something to stop you showing signs of an unpleasant deficiency disease is hardly the most imaginative or therapeutic way of establishing the level required for maximum health and efficiency. There do seem to be enormous variations. At one end of the scale we have therapists advising a gram or two a day, at the other we have

Linus Pauling talking about ten or even twenty grams in *Vitamin C and the common cold*.

Fortunately it is not possible to overdose on vitamin C in a way that would be dangerous. Because it is water soluble, excesses spill over into the urine. Some practitioners use a urine test to establish a dose for their patients, keeping them at a level where there is always a small excess. If the body is saturated with excess vitamin C then this may be reflected in loose bowel movements, so if you find you are getting diarrhoea then decrease your intake until these symptoms stop.

Knowing that you will excrete any vitamin C that you don't need means it is safe to start with a dose of 2 grams daily for a week or two. Gradually increase this according to your digestive tolerance. You could take up to six grams a day if you felt comfortable. Take vitamin C in divided doses, after meals, with water.

Ascorbic acid is the cheapest and the most widely available form of vitamin C. This is quite acceptable, but if you find it causes 'acidity' or digestive problems it might be as well to change to calcium ascorbate. Whenever possible take vitamin C with bio-flavonoids. These are co-agents that enhance the value of vitamin C and are often lost when it is produced synthetically. In the natural world the two are always found together. An orange for example contains vitamin C in the flesh and bio-flavonoids in the pith. Yet another reason for eating whole foods. In this respect, as in others, the whole orange is better than the extracted juice. Actually oranges are not the richest known source of vitamin C, just one of the most popular and convenient. Parsley, spinach and cabbage have a lot to offer, but not if it is all boiled away in the cooking process.

Vitamin C is very sensitive and is destroyed by

oxidation (i.e. exposure to air)

copper (watch out for kitchen utensils)

alkalis (baking powder)

pasteurizing (milk)
drying, water and heat (vegetables)
aspirin
smoking.

Looking at this list should be all the encouragement you need to take supplements. Add to it the fact that an editorial in the *BMJ* in 1976 referred to levels of vitamin C in leucocytes being lowered when the body is stressed. Obviously cancer patients are under a good deal of stress. Not just emotional stress either, some of the treatments for cancer are themselves stressful, and patients' needs would increase in these circumstances.

Dr Ewan Cameron claims some impressive responses from advanced cancer patients given very high doses of vitamin C (*National Medical Bulletin*, USA, September 1979). Unfortunately attempts to replicate his results have so far been unsuccessful.

Vitamin E

Tocopherol, usually alphatocopherol, a lipid soluble antioxidant that complements the action of vitamin C. Being fat soluble it can be stored for short periods in the body.

Uses Dr Evan Shute, author of *The Complete Updated Vitamin Book*, is a great enthusiast in the use of this vitamin for the control of cardiovascular disease. He claims that it decreases the oxygen requirements of muscles by as much as 43 per cent. It is its characteristic quality as a natural antioxidant that makes it particularly important to cancer patients. Cancer cells change from normal to embryonic form using fermentation, a process that is inhibited by the presence of oxygen. Perhaps because of its oxygenating effect, vitamin E has a reputation for enhancing healing and reducing scar tissue. There is some evidence that it may be involved in reproductive processes as well. Claims have been made for its power to improve the mobility of sperms in men and lessen the chances of miscarriage in women. Thus it is often associated with hormone activity and for this reason some therapists prefer not to give it to patients suffering from hormone-related cancers (typically breast, uterus, ovary). This reluctance is furthered by the possibility that vitamin E from natural vegetable sources might contain oestrogen as a contaminant. However, it is generally considered to be in the patients' interests to take vitamin E.

Dose A sensible dose would be 100iu daily, preferably emulsified in apple pectin to aid digestion. This dose should not create any problems but it should not be increased except under supervision because it is possible to build up unacceptably high levels. Like many vitamins, vitamin E is vulnerable to modern food processing methods. It is found in whole wheat and whole grains but not in refined, polished varieties of these foods.

Vitamin A

Vitamin A is one of a series of pigments called carotenes: alpha, beta, gamma etc. Beta-carotene is the one that converts most efficiently into vitamin A in the body, and it is known as a pro-vitamin.

Vitamin A is fat soluble and can be stored in the body. The liver is the main storage centre, and for this reason people suffering from liver disease are almost always deficient in vitamin A. The first signs of deficiency would probably be noticed in the eyes.

Uses The rods and cones of the retina of the eye are dependent on vitamin A and night blindness might be one of the first signs of deficiency. Known as the growth vitamin, it is essential for skeletal development. It also keeps the epithelial tissues (skin) healthy. Like other retinoids, vitamin A is believed to have a protective and therapeutic effect against certain cancers.

Dose It is difficult to establish a dose because some people have quantities of vitamin A already stored in the liver and available to them, others have none. It is possible to overdose on vitamin A, with serious consequences, so one should use both this substance and the carotenes, very carefully.

At Bristol our doctors advise taking carotene in the form of carrot juice. (All colourful vegetables, that have been pigmented yellow or green, contain carotene, but carrots lend themselves best to juicing.) If you drink more carotene than your body can convert, then the pigmentation will begin to show on your skin. The appearance of a slight yellow stain on the palms of the hands is likely to be the first sign of excess. At this point the dose should be reduced until normal colour returns. The carrot juice should be emulsified by whisking into it a teaspoonful of good quality oil. This will encourage it to circulate around the body in the bloodstream and not be sent to the liver for storage. Take 500–750 ml (1–1½ pints) of carrot juice daily.

Some people find the whole business of juicing very tedious. It is certainly a problem if you are out at work all day or cannot spare the money to buy a machine. In these circumstances beta-carotene capsules are ideal. Take one capsule containing 12,500iu beta-carotene twice a day.

Vitamin B

A group of the B vitamins is often included in the patient's programme because of their role in the general maintenance of health. They are not thought to be specifically active against cancer. This is a wide range of enzymes and co-enzymes that work together. It is more beneficial to take B vitamins in balanced formulation, but an excess of B12 and folic acid might not be in the cancer patient's interests.

B vitamins are water-soluble and excesses are excreted in urine and perspiration.

Uses   There are an enormous number of uses for these vitamins. They have an influence on the nervous system and are associated with stress relief, they play a role in the metabolism of food, and they are needed for the production of anti-bodies and red blood cells.

Bristol patients are advised to use brewer's yeast as the most acceptable form of B vitamins. This can be taken as a tablet or in powder form. The powder can be used as a flavour enhancer when sprinkled on to food. Some people find the yeast undigestible, especially if they are already suffering from extra wind from all the raw food. In this case we suggest they take a multi-B capsule. This might also be preferable for people who have too high a yeast population in their bodies already, women who suffer from thrush, for example.

Although widely available in modern diets these vitamins are vulnerable to

food processing
boiling (being water-soluble)
alcohol
sugar
certain drugs (i.e. some antibiotics)
the contraceptive pill

Dose   We recommend two tablets of high grade brewer's yeast taken three times daily. Brewer's yeast is also a good source of trace elements, especially chromium.

Selenium

Selenium is a trace element that acts as part of an anti-oxidant enzyme system. It is essential that it should be present in the body, but relatively small amounts are needed. It is usually present in the soil and taken up into our vegetables, but there are wide variations on maps showing where it is to be found that suggest this is not always the case. Glaciation seems to have had an adverse effect in the past, and current farming methods are doing no good in the present. The result is that there are areas (sometimes whole countries, like Finland) where selenium levels are very low.

The significance is that selenium deficiency has been shown to correlate with increased incidence of cancer in the population. One study showed that selenium deficiency could lead to a significant increase in the likelihood of developing cancer. (*BMJ* February 1985) See also Dr Richard Passwater's *Selenium as Food and Medicine*.

Uses   Taken together with vitamins C and E it contributes to a powerful anti-oxidant cocktail that is believed to be very helpful in the control of cancer. It is also protective against atherosclerosis, and helps in the functioning of the immune system generally. It is believed to be of considerable use in the prophylaxis of heart disease.

Dose   We recommend 200 mcg daily in an organic form.

It is difficult to know whether food contains selenium or not, consequently supplements are essential for cancer patients, but this dose should not be exceeded except under medical supervision.

Zinc

Another trace element, like selenium, that is not a major component of the body, but is rated as essential. This too has been leached out of the soil in glaciated areas and is adversely affected by chemicals in the soil.

Uses   It is involved in food metabolism. Retarded growth in general and of the sex organs in particular may indicate a deficiency. Its presence is essential for the effective action of certain enzymes involved in tissue healing and regeneration. It is present in leucocytes and is particularly important for patients suffering from leukaemia and lymphoma. Like selenium it is needed for the correct and full functioning of the immune system.

Dose   We recommend a starting dose of zinc orotate of 100 mg daily. This provides an elemental level of 16 mg of zinc.

These form the basis of the vitamin and mineral schedule recommended for patients at Bristol, but as far as possible these are tailored to meet individual requirements. We may also suggest additional supplements for certain individual cases.

Magnesium and **potassium** may be indicated. Low magnesium levels, like selenium, seem to correlate with increased cancer incidence in the population. Where levels are high in the soil, the incidence of cancer in the people is low. Together with potassium it has the effect of pushing out of the cells any excess sodium that may be interfering with normal cell function. The nutritional scheme we recommend is salt-free and high in potassium. This has the effect of reducing sodium and allowing more potassium to be taken up, and improved nutrition may be all that is needed to achieve this. But in severe cases it may be necessary to give supplements to encourage this process.

Although some of the vitamins and minerals listed here are cheap and freely available over the counter, if taken over a long period of time the business of shopping for them and paying for them becomes time-consuming and expensive. In the United Kingdom at the time of writing it is possible to have all these substances prescribed by a doctor and supplied through the National Health Service. This may take a while to set up, I must admit, because doctors are still somewhat confused over the recent regulations concerning what they can and cannot prescribe. a little gentle persuasion, and a reluctance to take 'no' for an answer will get you a long way. There are many patients coming to Bristol whose doctors willingly prescribe all their supplements without hesitation or difficulty. On the other hand some patients report that their doctors are under the impression that they are not allowed to do this.

Sometimes there are regional variations, but occasionally there can be differences in the same areas, even within a group practice itself where one doctor is prescribing and another is not. Usually this can be sorted out by means of a few telephone calls, but you may have to encourage your doctor by explaining that other patients are receiving their supplements in this way. Reluctance on the doctor's part is likely to be related to his anxiety that the bill for these things will one day end up on his desk. If he can talk to his colleagues and find out that this will not happen, he will probably be pleased to cooperate. By and large doctors will want to help you do all you can to help yourself. We have received, at Bristol, written confirmation from the Prescription Pricing Authority in Newcastle-upon-Tyne that these items can be ordered on the NHS and passed for payment by them.

Ever since the Cancer Help Centre began we have received invaluable help and support from

> Nature's Own Ltd
> 203–205 West Malvern Road
> West Malvern
> Worcs. WR14 4BB
> Tel: 06845 63465

This is a company that makes and supplies vitamins and minerals. They use the most natural sources they can and the safest methods of preparation possible. We use Nature's Own products at Bristol and the doctors who prescribe regularly for our patients usually specify that the products should come from them.

Because of their long association with the Cancer Help Centre they are familiar with the Bristol Programme and will answer any queries most willingly. They can also arrange for you to have a blood analysis done, and will supply everything you need for that.

Of course there are other companies that make and supply high-quality vitamins.

G. R. Lane Healthcrafts Ltd
Sissons Road
Gloucester GL1 3QB
Tel: 0452 24012

Nature's Best,
1 Lamberts Road
Tunbridge Wells
Kent TN2 3EQ Tel: 0892 34143

Nutricare Ltd (Gerrard House)
736 Christchurch Road
Bournemouth
Tel: 0202 35352.

There is such a great, and rising, interest in the use of supplements that stores are full of wholesome-looking packages promising everything from healthy hair to pain-free periods. Shop around until you find what suits you, but read the labels carefully. Check the quantities – the actual amount contained in each capsule. Some of these products are overpriced and sugar-coated. You don't want either of these things. The people who own and run health-food stores and pharmacies where vitamins and minerals are usually on sale are likely to be well-informed and helpful, but whenever possible get professional advice.

COMPLEMENTARY SUPPLEMENTS

There are some additional therapies that we do NOT use at Bristol, but are still the subject of great interest to our patients. This may be because we have at one time included them in our programme – amygdalin for example – or because we often recommend patients to seek these treatments elsewhere: this would be true of iscador. A few lines here might be of interest, and help readers to expand the holistic model in ways that appeal to them.

Amygdalin

Otherwise known as laetrile or B17, this is a substance extracted from apricot kernels and other natural food sources. Mention of it can be guaranteed to raise a riot of feeling, both for and against. This is a substance that has caused passions to run high, and many a legal battle has been fought over it. Some practitioners in other countries have gone to gaol in defiance of government bans concerning its use. In America it has been banned in many states at the insistence of the Federal Drug Authority.

Advocates of amygdalin say:

It has been suppressed for political reasons.

It is in the vested interests of the drug companies to prevent the use of something so freely available and inexpensive.

Because of this, amygdalin has never been given a fair trial and proper tests.

The antagonists say:

Desperate, very sick people must be protected from exploitation by the self-interest of the people who manufacture and administer amygdalin.

That it doesn't have any therapeutic value, and tests show this.

Not very helpful.

In the absence of more satisfactory data it would normally be wise to 'wait and see' but there are two reasons why amygdalin might be worth a try. The first is that there are well-documented cases of hundreds of patients who claim to have been cured by it. The second is that, properly administered, it appears to be harmless. Obviously the antagonists would dispute both of these statements but I was impressed by information I received from Ernesto Contreras in Mexico, a doctor who has used amygdalin for many years. I have visited his clinic in Tijuana where he has treated tens of thousands of cancer patients with high doses of amygdalin, none of whom, he says, has ever suffered any negative side-effects. He places great store by the value of amygdalin in his therapeutic programme, but it must be remembered that it is only a part of the therapy he uses. This exceptional physician incorporates diet, supplements, counselling, prayer and healing into the patient's regime. In such circumstances it would be difficult to isolate the value of amygdalin, but when he tells me he has never seen toxic side-effects, I believe him. If amygdalin only works in conjunction with other holistic therapies anyone following the Bristol programme would be a good candidate for it.

The reason amygdalin is sometimes called vitamin B17 is because some people believe it to be essential to health and normal growth. It is found in the pips and kernels of apples, apricots, grapes, peaches, plums and other fruit, and in certain grains, like millet. Thus it can claim to be a natural nutrient, and its presence in the diet has been given as an explanation for why certain groups of people, like the Hunzas and the Pueblo Indians, have lower incidences of cancer than we do. Because there are so many other reasons why these people are not as vulnerable to cancer as the rest of us, I personally think it is naïve to attach too much importance to the role of amygdalin in isolation. And even if it does have an important preventive role, when it comes to using this substance as a therapy, when cancer is already present, we have to do much more than eat it.

Actually we should be wary of eating too much of it at any time. The enthusiastic ingestion of cupfuls of apple-pips and handfuls of apricot kernels is dangerous. It is almost certainly as a result of misguided misuse that cases of toxic overdose have been reported. There is a cyanide molecule present in amygdalin which might be released in the stomach when mixed with digestive juices, so one should limit the number of kernels that are eaten in isolation from the fruits that contain them. The idea is to get the cyanide to release at the site of the cancer cells, and the efficient way to do this is to by-pass the stomach and pour the amygdalin straight into the bloodstream. The best way of doing this is via intravenous injections.

Obviously this requires the support and cooperation of your doctor.

In view of the bad press that amygdalin has received over the years, this cooperation may be in short supply. If all he has read is the write-up in the *New Scientist* (Sept. 1978) of a report in the *New England Journal of Medicine* (vol 299, 1978) then your doctor is entitled to be less than enthusiastic. Perhaps if he knew that when practitioners were invited to submit their experiences of using amygdalin its use was actually illegal, he might feel that this was less than a fair trial, and be less influenced by its luke-warm findings.

An account of some of the long history of bitterness and debate that has surrounded this substance is given by G. Edward Griffen in his book *World Without Cancer – the story of vitamin B17*. One glance at the title will tell you that this is not an unbiased view, but it is a fascinating and informative read.

More information can be had from Nature's Own. They have been supplying amygdalin to doctors for many years and will answer any queries about it.

If time and money allow, then a visit to the Centro Clinico del Mar in Mexico would take you to a place with almost unprecedented experience in the use of this substance. Their mailing address is P.O. Box 1561, Chula Vista, California 92012.

Iscador

Iscador is a substance extracted from mistletoe. This has long been considered to be a magical plant with healing powers, but it was the work of Rudolph Steiner that led to its use in this form. Iscador is an anthroposophical medicine and is best prescribed by a doctor who has been trained in the anthroposophical method. A list of these doctors can be obtained from:

Rudolph Steiner House,
35 Park Road
London NW1 6XT.

Also, The Royal Homoeopathic Hospital, Great Ormond Street, London WC1N 3HT, has been very accommodating and helpful to some of our patients in relation to the use of iscador.

During the initial consultation the doctor will decide how you should take the iscador, the mixture and strength of the dose, and the frequency. This varies from person to person, but once established it tends to stay the same, and patients may continue with the same routine for many years. Sometimes one or two consultations with the anthroposophical doctor will be all you need. He can then write to your own doctor and explain what he has advised you to do. Your own doctor can prescribe iscador on the National Health Service.

Sometimes iscador is taken by mouth, but more often it is injected. You can always ask your doctor to give these injections, and I have heard of patients who are visited by their district nurse for this purpose. But these are simple subcutaneous injections that you can easily learn to give yourself, and this allows you more freedom and independence.

Iscador has been extensively tested in Europe and has been shown to have beneficial effects on a great many different cancers at varying stages of development. It seems to work by initiating an immunological response, and patients may experience a slight rise in temperature. Since fever is considered to be a favourable response, this is usually welcomed. Its use is frequently attended by a significant increase in lymphocytes which the body can put to good use in its defence against cancer.

An anthroposophical doctor talking to me about iscador said, 'It reminds the body who its enemies are.' Since cancer patients are playing host to a parasite that will kill them if left unchecked, a reminder of this sort would be welcome and timely.

COMPLEMENTARY THERAPIES

Acupuncture

I don't think it is just the fact that I am an acupuncturist that explains the consistent interest among Bristol patients in this particular branch of Chinese medicine. Acupuncture has enjoyed a great deal of publicity and popularity in recent years in relation to its success in the treatment of a wide range of common disorders. Quite understandably people wonder if it would help them in the fight against cancer.

The traditional Chinese model of disease is entirely holistic, seeing treatment always in terms of mind, body and spirit. In this respect acupuncture blends well with the Bristol Programme, and I think it has a part to play in the overall treatment of cancer patients, but we should not have naïve expectations of it. The fact that acupuncture can be dramatically and instantaneously effective in the treatment of hay fever, for example, does not mean that it can dissolve tumours overnight. However, it can improve your capacity to heal yourself. Adjustments to the flow of your energy can have far-reaching effects on your physical performance.

While I was staying in Issels' clinic in Bavaria I was visited by an acupuncture colleague of mine, Dr Evans. Josef Issels took him on his ward rounds and discussed the patients with him. He asked Dr Evans if he could treat a girl in her mid-twenties who was suffering from leukaemia, and not making very good progress despite all of his attentions and the full gamut of conventional treatment. Issels was able to assess the value of the acupuncture on the basis of feedback from blood tests done in his laboratory. It seemed to him that the acupuncture treatment was bringing about changes in the composition of the girl's blood and she decided to continue treatment after she left the clinic.

Nobody would say that acupuncture should be used alone in the treatment of cancer – least of all the Chinese – but as a complementary therapy it can be very helpful. I have known it to be of great help with post-operative pain, especially when surgery has interfered with the flow of energy by cutting across the channels through which it would normally pass. This would usually be a self-righting mechanism, but sometimes the body is slow to readjust after the trauma of surgical incisions, with the result that patients suffer unnecessary discomfort that a good acupuncturist could relieve.

In many countries, the United Kingdom included, anyone can practise acupuncture. They don't need a qualification, just a packet of needles and a book or two. Obviously you must be careful whom you allow to treat you, because, if not administered properly, it can do you harm as well as good.

There is a register of British Acupuncturists that is published by the Council for Acupuncture. Copies are available on request from:

British Acupuncture Association and Register
34 Alderney Street
London SW1V 4EU

Register of Traditional Chinese Medicine
7a Thorndean Street
London SW18 4HE

Traditional Acupuncture Society
11 Grange Park
Stratford-upon-Avon
Warwickshire CV37 6XH
(A joint register of practitioners can be obtained from this last address.)

Once you have established that your local practioner is qualified, then make a few enquiries and talk to someone who has been treated there. There are a lot of part-time practitioners who lack experience and it would be good to know this if possible. If your nearest acupuncturist lives fifty miles away, think again. You would almost certainly need a course of treatment, going weekly to begin with and then gradually expanding the interval between visits. There is a limit to how much time, money and energy one can reasonably invest in just one aspect of an holistic programme. It might be more sensible to focus attention on something more readily accessible.

Homoeopathy

Like acupuncture, this system of healing is based on the principle of treating the whole person and would fit in well to a holistic scheme. I have met homoeopaths who have claimed to have cured cancer using their methods and none other, but I would not advocate this route alone. Every system of medicine will have its successes, and, quite understandably, practitioners dwell on these and gloss over the failures. When a therapy is not invasive and dangerous I think it is worth trying, especially since there are almost certain to be benefits, even when it cannot claim to cure.

Homoeopathy works on the principle of 'like cures like' and is based on the work of Samuel Hahnemann. He experimented with using minute dilutions of various substances to treat the symptoms that those same substances would give rise to if taken in larger doses. Arsenic, for example, causes the body to erupt with diarrhoea and vomiting and the fear of imminent death. Anyone who has suffered from acute food poisoning will know just how this feels. I for one have cause to be grateful both for Hahnemann and the fact that most French chemists stock arsenicum album which can have an almost miraculously soothing effect on this condition.

Make enquiries about qualified practitioners from:

The British Homoeopathic Association
27a Devonshire Street
London W1N 1RJ

The Homoeopathic Trust
Hahnemann House
2 Powis Place
Great Ormond Street
London WC1N 3HT

There are homoeopathic hospitals in London and some other cities where advice would also be forthcoming.

Some homoeopaths did not start out life as medical doctors, so they are trained homoeopaths but not registered doctors. A list of these practitioners can be obtained from:

Society of Homoeopaths
2a Bedford Place
Southampton
Hants SO1 2BY

After the initial consultation and a few follow-up visits it is often possible to continue treatment at home with only occasional visits to the practitioner.

Books on homoeopathy make fascinating reading. One that would particularly interest breast cancer patients is the chapter entitled 'Phytolacca' in *The Physician's Posy* by D. R. Blackie.

Herbalism

The use of herbs and plants for their curative value is one of the oldest of all methods of healing. However, there is a bit more to it than drinking herb teas. Some of the compounds used are highly complex, and you should make sure you are in the hands of a properly qualified practitioner. If the idea appeals to you, contact:

The National Institute of Medical Herbalists
41 Hatherley Road
Winchester
Hampshire SO22 6RR

The General Council and Register of Consultant Herbalists
Marlborough House
Swanpool
Falmouth
Cornwall TR11 4HW

Rather like homoeopathy, after the initial consultation you will be taking a remedy at home and returning for check-ups.

Naturopathy

Naturopaths are often trained also as osteopaths, but it is their skill in the realms of diet and natural healing that you need. I think it is best to steer clear of osteopathy while there is cancer active in the body.

If you are lucky enough to have a good naturopath nearby she could be very helpful to you. In the chapter on nutrition I stressed that diet is a very personal affair and should, ideally, be tailored to fit individual requirements. A naturopath would be just the person to do this for you; to establish your best vitamin and mineral regime. They will probably know a lot about posture and breathing which would also be helpful.

British Naturopathic and Osteopathic Association
6 Netherhall Gardens
London NW3 5RR

A register of members is available from:
The Secretary
Slaters
5 Guildford Road
Broadbridge Heath
Horsham
West Sussex RH12 3JF

Summary

Having established that a practitioner is qualified, do not be afraid to ring up and talk about your situation. It is very important that you should feel comfortable and confident with the person you see. Important too that he or she should have plenty of experience. Many practitioners are using their healing skills on a part-time basis and may never have treated a cancer patient before. You need to be with someone who will understand about the diet you are on and relate knowledgeably to the effect of the various vitamins and minerals you are taking. If you raise these matters before making your first appointment you will stand a better chance of finding the best person to treat you. Not all alternative practitioners are holistic in their outlook, and you need someone like this when you are trying to put the Bristol Programme into effect.

Many doctors take up alternative medicine and practise it alongside their usual more traditional techniques. On the face of it this might sound ideal, but although they may be wonderful doctors, they still may not have the skill you require. Doctors who are members of

The British Holistic Medical Association
179 Gloucester Place
London NW1 6DX

are more likely to be working in the way you need. Contact them and ask for advice.

3

Mind Over Matter

MACBETH   Canst thou not minister to a mind diseas'd,
              Pluck from the memory a rooted sorrow,
              Raze out the written troubles of the brain,
              And with some sweet oblivious antidote
              Cleanse the stuff'd bosom of that perilous stuff
              Which weighs upon the heart?
DOCTOR   Therein the patient
              Must minister to himself.

Macbeth, Act V, scene 3

STRESS IN RELATION TO DISEASE

Nice try Macbeth, nice try.

Soon after their arrival at Bristol patients will have a private session with a counsellor. They will also share in group learning the practice of stress control techniques.

Who has not longed at some time or another for some 'sweet oblivious antidote' to our troubles? Judging by the tons of tranquillizers, anti-depressants and sleeping pills we consume, to say nothing of the alarming rise of the use of so-called 'recreational' drugs, an ever-increasing number of us are finding our lives more than we can cope with. How much longer are we going to look outside of ourselves for solutions?

The doctor's blunt, uncompromising reply to Macbeth may not appear a very helpful answer on the surface of it, but he knew just as surely as Macbeth himself that Lady Macbeth was sick from a cause that no medicine or potion could cure.

Her problems were such that she had to deal with them herself and not look to another to come up with a patent remedy.

Which one of us has not at some time wished we could find a way to 'pluck out a rooted sorrow'? Who hasn't been plagued by 'the written troubles of the brain' or felt the weight of 'that perilous stuff' heavy on our hearts? We all know how deeply we can be affected by our emotions and how difficult it is sometimes to stop feeling sad or angry long after the occasion for it has passed.

After a television interview years ago in which I said I believed that my cancer was stress-related, we were swamped at Bristol by people who also felt like that. One of our first patients was a women who thought that her guilt and anxiety concerning the suffering of her anorexic daughter was the reason behind her cancer. She was almost hysterical with relief at being able to express how she felt. She described how she went for hospital visits feeling inside her that it was all a waste of time, that a woman who had failed as a mother deserved to die. She said, 'I almost felt guilty having the treatment because I didn't believe it would ever work for me, and I was just wasting everyone's time and money.'

I shall repeat many times that the issue in such a case is not so much whether this woman was right about any of this, but that she *believed* she was right. Knowing what we know about the deleterious effect of stress on the immune system she may in fact have been close to the truth, but in any event, she was in the worst possible frame of mind to benefit from hospital treatment.

Most of us have been close enough to experiences of mental stress and anxiety to know that it is possible, quite literally, to make ourselves ill with worry. Quite frequently, in everyday life, we find ourselves observing that a friend who has had 'flu three times this year has 'been under a lot of pressure lately'. We are quite happy about accepting a correlation between stress and minor health disorders and we should not be afraid of looking at the possible role of mental stress in relation to much more serious illnesses. In the case of Lady Macbeth her guilt and fear drove her to madness and ultimate suicide, and I have known many who believe anxiety played a part in the breakdown of health that led to the development of cancer. For as long as doctors have kept records they have been observing a relationship between cancer and the mental disposition of the patient. So we should be open to this possibility. As far back as the second century Galen had observed that 'melancholic' women were more likely to get breast cancer than 'sanguine' women.

Before expanding on the relationship between mental stress and cancer it is most important to make clear that there is no automatic and direct causal connection. I am not implying that everyone who gets cancer is covering up some inner pain and suffering. This is quite obviously not the case, and no one should feel they are under some kind of pressure to pick away at their emotions and feelings until they come up with something that could qualify as a causative stress factor. It is bad enough having cancer in the first place without then having to put up with someone suggesting it is all your fault and you brought it on yourself because you are such a neurotic. Mental and emotional stress is not an automatic precursor to the development of cancer. However, just as it is ridiculous and unfair for people to feel cornered into unnecessary self-analysis it is not right for other people to be denied their belief that anxiety has made them ill. Some people will not have to ponder for long on whether fear, grief or any other emotional stress has been instrumental in the breakdown of their health: they will know immediately. One of our counsellors at Bristol believes that for some people this may be the case, but they are not aware of it. She says, 'Some of the deepest wounds can seemingly take months or years to surface, yet are festering busily in the subconscious all the time.' Such a person might need help to access this deeply buried suffering.

It is in the nature of things that people who do feel there has been an emotional component in the breakdown of their health are likely to find their way to us in Bristol. Consequently the fact that a very high percentage of our patients feel this way does not necessarily mirror the feelings of cancer patients as a whole. Many people lead stressful and emotional lives and cope perfectly well.

If you are pretty sure that your stress management techniques are good and that you are not burdened with unresolved anxiety you will probably have left this chapter to read until last of all, but please do read it. It is tempting to fall into the way of thinking that says, 'If you damaged your immune system by feeding yourself carelessly, then diet is the answer' or 'If you think your cancer is stress-related, then counselling is the thing.' This kind of thinking can be helpful in narrowing the field a bit when starting out on the task of putting together an anti-cancer regime, but we should quickly expand into as many areas as possible or we shall miss a great deal. If you consider yourself such a cool, laid-back person that you never learn to meditate, you are depriving yourself of an immensely useful technique. So, even if you don't identify with Macbeth's desperate plea to the doctor, read on, you might learn something interesting.

A physician called Sir James Paget observed a hundred years ago that: 'The cases are so frequent in which deep anxiety, deferred hope and disappointment are quickly followed by the growth and increase of cancer, that we can hardly doubt that mental depression is a weighty additive to the other influences favouring the development of the cancerous constitution.'

Although from as long ago as Galen's time it has been noticed and recorded regularly by doctors that cancer is often associated with certain mental dispositions, observations of these aspects of the disease are found less frequently in nineteenth-century medical texts. It was then that the use of ether and other forms of anaesthesia became regular practice, enabling doctors to perform operations on inert and peaceful patients who were not writhing in pain. This naturally enlarged their scope considerably and, most understandably, made way for an increased interest in surgery and surgical techniques, so the emotional and mental aspects of health and disease took a back seat for a while. But they are re-emerging now, as never before, as factors demanding serious attention.

It is not yet clear exactly *how* our immune system is affected by stress but that it *is* affected has been shown time and again. The most experienced researcher on this subject is Dr Hans Selye and he has written at length on the subject. His books *The Stress of Life* and *Stress without Distress* are worth referring to.

A study by Dr Holmes and Dr Rahe at Washington Medical School involved the use of a 'social re-adjustment scale' to predict the likelihood of disease. The scale worked on a points system, some stress factors scoring more than others. Holmes and Rahe showed that the probability of being ill correlated closely with the number of points each individual scored. In other words, if you had been having a bad time of it lately, then you were more likely to fall sick. Of course you knew that already, didn't you? Some of this is so painfully obvious it is embarrassing and insulting to the patient that so little notice is taken of it. When did *your* doctor last suggest that you might not have to come and see him so often if you learned a good stress control technique? To give credit where it's due, one of my most prized possessions is a prescription pad on which my own doctor wrote the name of a book of meditation exercises. We're getting there.

Identifying what's going on

Let us suppose that you do have something troubling you deeply. You may or may not feel that this has been a contributory factor in your illness, that doesn't matter. If something is weighing on your mind it is affecting your well-being and will stand in the way of you achieving a peaceful balanced existence, which is the precursor to good health.

Some experiences in life hit us so hard that we continue to react to them for many years afterwards. For example, if we are made redundant after years of faithful service, it would be natural to feel resentful and angry and insecure and frightened. These are not inappropriate feelings and it is important that we should express them at the time. Indeed, being able to express them properly may be the key towards letting them go. But sometimes we continue to feel angry and resentful long afterwards, even when we have found, and settled into, a new job. We may find that although we stop feeling insecure and frightened because we are now earning good money and have excellent pension rights, we are still harbouring anger and resentment. We may find it impossible to expunge the way we were made to feel by the experience of the redundancy even when it is a thing of the past. We may even justify the continuance of our emotional response with remarks like, 'I can forgive, but I can't forget' or, inevitably, 'I can forget but I can't forgive'. The truth is we can't do either. We are still being poisoned by these feelings and don't know how to get rid of them.

This can apply to just about any experience you care to name. When my parents died I felt a terrible sense of loss; I grieved and I mourned and I cried a lot. This was perfectly acceptable behaviour for someone who saw herself orphaned within the space of nine weeks; however, it would be a funny way to be carrying on now, eight years later. Even so I have met people who continue to grieve the loss of someone precious for the whole of the rest of their lives. They justify this with remarks like, 'I just can't forget her' or, 'Nobody will ever be able to replace him'. The fact is, we shouldn't be trying to forget or replace, but we are in such an emotional muddle we don't know what we should be doing, never mind how to do it. We may need help. I think the person most likely to help in this situation – or anything remotely like it – is a counsellor.

COUNSELLING

Inevitably this word has overtones of advice and guidance, implying that a counsellor will tell us what to do. This is not always the case, although it may be. Sometimes counsellors say very little, but you find that when you are with them they help you to see what it is you want to do, what you yourself feel is best.

Many people have some inbuilt resistance to the idea of going for counselling. I think this comes from the belief that somehow one ought not to need help, it ought to be possible to sort things out for oneself. There is a delicate balance between helping oneself and looking for help from other people, but turning for outside help can be a very important part of any self-development process. One of our therapists at Bristol says that admitting we need help is the first step on the road to autonomy.

What might we expect from a course of counselling?

Even if we are not already carrying an emotional load before falling ill, it would be a most unusual person who could hear that they have cancer without getting pretty upset about it. Obviously not everyone falls to pieces, but I did, and I hear weekly stories of others who did as well. The tremendous uprush of emotions that engulfed me at the time, and that were never far away for months afterwards, did in fact puzzle me rather. In my saner, quieter moments I tried to analyse what was making me so upset and came to the conclusion that it was what Elizabeth Khubler-Ross calls 'unfinished business'. I took this little lot to a counsellor. With her help I dared to look at the parts of my life that I felt I had been making a mess of, either because they felt too painful to expose or because I felt inadequate to deal with them properly. For the first time in years I stopped feeling a guilty, anxious failure. This meant I had a lot less 'perilous stuff' weighing on my heart, leaving room for other more healing and creative thoughts. I was also able to express my feelings about dying, my fears for the children, my sisters, my husband – things that are not easy to talk through with someone too close, because they too need to talk about their reactions to your illness.

Many people who are keen on self-help therapies feel that you should be able to manage without counselling. Of course, some people manage perfectly well without it, but if we feel we must always do everything to help ourselves and never reach out to others for their assistance it may be that our personality and up-bringing is working against us. If we think that getting help from outside is a sign of weakness it might take quite a bit of courage to make that first appointment with a counsellor. I actually found it easier to cope with some tough and painful physical cancer treatments than pick up the phone and agree to talk about things I had kept locked away inside myself for years. But once I had started nothing could stop me. Counselling can be a very challenging encounter, but it can also be soothing, stimulating, exciting and comforting. A good counsellor will enable you to identify your problems.

I am never upset for the reason I think

If we peel away the layers and have a look at what is really causing the disturbance, we may find that it has no hold over us any more. The woman still angry about her redundancy may find that it wasn't the loss of the job that allowed these feelings of resentment to become part of her life. She may find that she has always tended towards feelings like this towards the world and the experience of losing her job brought this tendency sharply into focus and gave her an excuse to feel the way she always wanted to feel.

Why would anyone want to feel angry and resentful all the time? Lots of reasons. Most likely this is a learned response from childhood experiences that is triggered off over and over again throughout life, causing reaction rather than action under stress. If this kind of situation is relevant to us we may find that just knowing what's going on is enough to put it right.

But what if identifying the problem doesn't go anywhere near to resolving it?

Do you need to change the situation or your reaction to it?

This is an important question. We often tell ourselves we can't do anything when in fact we can. The reason we don't act is because we are too frightened of the consequences.

Time and again people say to me, 'I know exactly what my problem is, I just can't do anything about it.' I sympathize because I felt exactly the same. I thought I knew why I had cancer, I could identify the problem very clearly, but if I had known how to cope with it I would have done so already and wouldn't have ended up in hospital. I felt like a hamster in a wheel, running round to the same place all the time and never getting anywhere.

I had managed to convince myself that there was nothing I could do because I had not entertained the possibility that I could change. It never occurred to me that I could become the sort of person who *could* cope with the problems that were sending me to the wall. I could change and I did change. So can you.

Just as a matter of interest I wrote my first book in an attempt to show how helpless, incoherent, confused, depressed, uncertain and unstable I used to be. I spent so much of my time explaining to patients at Bristol that I used to be an impoverished, nervous little wimp and then changed gradually into something different, I decided to write about the process of making those changes. This has cheered everybody up no end. Having read about the muddle I was in before I got cancer, patients know that, even if they feel like that now, it is possible to change and grow stronger. So, if you are struggling with the emotional impact of a situation that you cannot change, don't feel that this rules out any possibility of dealing with its effect on you.

But we should not immediately rule out the possibility of

changing the situation. This may be the quickest and most effective way of relieving ourselves of a great deal of stress. Even if right now you feel too weak or too scared to do anything, it is possible to acquire the strength and resilience you need to make important changes. One of our patients was carrying the burden of looking after an elderly relative and this was exhausting her emotionally and physically. It turned out that it was her own poor self-image and lack of confidence that had created the situation where it was hard for her to ask for the help she needed and deserved. She just couldn't face the unpleasantness and criticism that she thought would be the consequence of asking her brothers and sisters to do their share. As it turned out, the rest of the family was happy to help, but had always been intimidated by her efficiency and assumed she wanted to be in charge.

A good counsellor can help us look at our view of ourselves, why we think people are looking for excuses not to like us, why we find it hard not to be liked, what stops us standing up for our rights. They may also show us ways of getting our needs met that we have never thought of before. My counsellor helped me to jump off the wheel of helplessness and start behaving in a more purposeful way. I found that there were things I could change without drama or damage.

For many years now doctors and therapists treating cancer patients have been observing certain characteristics that many of them seem to have in common. One of these is to do with having difficulty in expressing negative emotions, and more is said about this later in this book. When I first read that I was quite indignant because I was a great protestor and defender of human rights. I could and did get quite worked up in the name of causes and movements. What I couldn't do was get worked up about my own rights. In this respect I shared a quality that I have seen time and again in cancer patients: I was very good at meeting other people's needs but very poor at attending to my own. Very often we become so caught up in looking after other people and making sure they are happy, well fed and fulfilled, we lose sight of what we want for ourselves.

Lawrence Le Shan's poignant phrase 'singing your own song' (see Suggested reading, page 131) describes perfectly what I am referring to here. Do we have a proper balance between serving other people and serving ourselves?

Have we allowed our lives to become so crowded by pressures from outside that there is no time or space for us to 'sing our own song'? Are we afraid that we couldn't do it if we tried? Or scared that someone would stop us? Have we so lost touch with ourselves that we hardly know any longer what our song really is? Once I would have had to answer 'yes' to all these questions, but I wouldn't now. That's what counselling can do for you.

RELAXATION AND MEDITATION

If we have to allow that there may be situations that could be changed if *we* changed, then we must also allow that there are some situations that cannot be changed. You may be burdened with the care of an elderly relative and *not* have anyone you can turn to for help: whatever I do I can never bring my parents back to life; children crippled by thalidomide cannot grow new arms and legs. Sometimes when faced with situations that we cannot control, we give up all together. We recognize that we are going to have to learn to live with the situation, but we very rarely do – learn to *live* with it I mean. We often learn to resent it, learn to hate it, learn to be dispirited and broken by it, but few of us learn how to continue to live a meaningful and fulfilling life in the face of suffering.

This is hardly surprising since we have been taught that suffering is bad, that it is something that should not be allowed, and that it is always a disaster. Not all cultures share this belief. Indeed it is somewhat surprising that we think like this, since our word 'suffer' also means 'permit' or 'tolerate'.

Jesus talked about 'suffering the little children to come unto Him' and we refer to 'not suffering fools gladly' and in both cases we mean allow. I think we would get along a lot better with coping with suffering if we could accept it. Suffering is part of the way things are. Sometimes we can make it go away, sometimes we cannot. Living in a society that insists we must make it go away has weakened our mechanisms for coping with it. It is possible to learn how to handle better those situations which cannot be changed. Just as it might be necessary for us to learn how to become strong enough to leap into action and start altering the world about us when that is possible, so is it also necessary for us to learn new ways of handling stressful situations that we cannot change. Counselling can help with this too.

If you are wondering what all this has to do with cancer, the connection is stress. When we feel frustrated and see no end to our disappointment we are experiencing stress just as surely as the teenager facing important examinations or the mother mourning her still-born child. Stress may be chronic or acute, but, unless we have mechanisms for coping with it, it will have an unhealthy effect on us.

To try and clarify the picture a bit it might help to say that emotional stress may be best dealt with by a counsellor, but the physical effects that emotional stress can have is dealt with through relaxation or meditation. You may need to keep reminding yourself that thoughts and feelings in your mind transmit themselves into physical bio-chemical changes in the body, but as long as this is only a temporary experience then the stress should not harm us.

We must be clear about this: there is nothing wrong with stress providing it doesn't last for ever. If we know how to recover from it and let it pass we protect ourselves from damage. If we know how to bounce back after being knocked down, if we know how to leave the office worries behind and relax at the end of the day, if we know when enough is enough and bow out of everything by taking a holiday, then we are not likely to be victims to the negative aspects of stress.

Remember there are positive aspects too. One man's stress is another man's excitement. What exhausts one person stimulates another. Wonderful things like dancing, winning at roulette and making love can be stressful, but they are also very enjoyable. It makes no sense to say that these things are bad in themselves, but I wouldn't be at all surprised if just as many people have dropped dead with a heart attack in the casino or in bed, as on the squash court or at the office. Knowing the difference between stress and distress is an important prerequisite for health.

Ainslie Meares, an Australian doctor and psychiatrist and an expert in the use of altered states of consciousness in the control of cancer, believed that many people have become so used to stress that their first experience of deep relaxation comes as quite a shock. This is the view, too, of Dr Herbert Benson, author of *The Relaxation Response* who uses stress control as part of his programme for patients suffering from high blood pressure. He says that people think they are relaxing simply because they have dropped a degree or two of their tenseness. This suggests that we are severely out of touch with our relaxation response but have a dangerous familiarity with chronic levels of stress. The worrying thing about all this is that stress triggers off the 'fight or flight' response in the autonomic nervous system. This means that all sorts of things could be going on in our bodies that may be inappropriate and dangerous, but we are not aware of this.

Man is constructed in such a way that the roar of a wild bear or the sound of a fire alarm bell will start a chain reaction of responses that improve his chances of either defending himself or escaping: in other words, fighting or fleeing from danger. If our lives are threatened then we need immediate and special help. This is given in the form of hormone secretions – steroids and adrenalin – released from the adrenal cortex, with dramatic effects in the body. The flow of blood to the brain is increased so you can make best use of what wits you have, and the flow of blood to the skin is reduced so you won't lose too much blood if you are wounded, and there is more blood to power your muscles for action. Digestive acids flow into the stomach in order to release as much sugar as possible into the bloodstream to raise potential energy levels. At the same time there is an increase in the heart beat, raised blood pressure, relaxation of airways and deeper, more energetic breathing. This is all very helpful indeed if you are fighting bears or escaping from burning buildings. Unfortunately this often happens when we open the gas bill and don't have the money to pay it, or get stuck in a traffic jam when we are already late for work. We may react so stressfully to these situations that we trigger off the fight or flight response when we can neither fight nor flee. Instead the stress simmers away inside us, unreleased. Or does it? Do we have to become one of those archetypes of anxiety with a sweaty face, a nervous twitch and permanently high blood pressure? No we don't.

Lots of people are subjected to considerable stresses and strains but appear to be none the worse for it. Whenever I talk about cancer as a stress-related disease someone always asks me nervously if I think they will get cancer, because they have just suffered a bereavement or they have a very stressful job. There is no reason to suppose they will necessarily fall ill, with cancer or anything else, because a healthy, well adjusted body will not stay stressed for ever. We are not designed to maintain the fight or flight 'red alert' situation for long periods of time, and when the danger or stress is passed, the body systems quieten down and everything returns to normal. At least that is what should happen, and when it does we can safely say that stress has done no more than evoke a natural and normal response in the body which has now passed. Unfortunately there are some people who do not recover from stress in this way, they stay tensed even when the situation does not demand it, and this is harmful to their health.

So many of us have adapted to chronically high levels of

stress that we now assume a state of stress to be 'normal'. We are so used to being tense we have forgotten how it feels to be relaxed. One of the first things we must re-learn if we are to start being healthy again is how to relax.

For the purposes of discussion I am making a distinction between relaxation and meditation. Obviously these two activities overlap and blur into each other, but it is as well to remember that it is possible to relax the body thoroughly while the mind is buzzing away, busy with thoughts. People who say they relax in front of the television are doing something like this – relaxing their bodies but not their minds.

Relaxation

Bristol devotes a lot of time to the teaching of relaxation techniques. This is because we share the belief that people have to be re-educated in how to relax. Every day begins and ends with a half-hour session led by a member of staff. This gives patients the benefit of a variety of approaches and styles, allowing them to experience several different ways of relaxing. It also helps them to establish regular relaxation sessions as a part of their daily routine.

There are also specific times during the week when the staff who are specialists in the teaching of these techniques talk them through and explain them to patients. This enables people to ask questions and raise any difficulties they may be having during the twice daily sessions.

Something that crops up time and again is the question 'How do I know if I am really relaxed? Can I be sure I'm doing it properly?' We are fortunate at Bristol to have therapists who are familiar with the work of Dr Schultz and Dr Luthe in relation to autogenic training. This is an excellent training and is highly recommended (an address for obtaining more information is given at the end of the chapter). The state of relaxation achieved through autogenic training is characterized by feelings of warmth and heaviness, saliva in the mouth, calm regular breathing, and no rapid eye movements. The first of these signs patients can be aware of for themselves and they are ways of knowing that they are achieving deep levels of relaxation. Another way of finding how relaxed you are would be to use bio-feedback techniques.

Bio-feedback   A bio-feedback machine is the name given to a piece of equipment that tells you about something happening in your body that you could not otherwise know. A thermometer tells you how high or low your temperature is; a sphygmometer tells you what your blood pressure is. These are both examples of bio-feedback equipment.

If you are trying to learn relaxation techniques then it is sometimes quite useful to know how you are getting on. At Bristol we use bio-feedback machines that monitor skin resistance and show when you are completely relaxed. You just strap a metal contact to the palm of your hand; this is attached by a wire to a little black box which is placed on the table in front of you. There is a dial on the box that shows a needle moving to the right if you are excited or tense and to the left if you are relaxed and peaceful.

There are many different machines on the market. Some are very complicated and expensive and offer a screen positively popping with information in the form of flashing lights, but these are best used under supervision. It is not always easy to interpret all the data and anyway you have to have your eyes open in order to do so. Deep relaxation is sometimes quite difficult to achieve and it is harder still with your eyes open. Other machines give feedback about your state of consciousness by emitting soft bleeps of sound. This has the advantage of allowing you to keep your eyes closed, but some people find themselves tensing in anticipation of the sound, which is the exact opposite of what you want to achieve. Our choice of the Skin Resistance Meter was based on the fact that it is cheap and very simple to use. It only requires you to open your eyes at the end of the session and make a note of what has happened to the needle.

Because there are so many ways of learning to relax or meditate, some patients find it helpful to use a bio-feedback machine in order to see which works best for them. Some people may find that certain mental images have a profoundly relaxing effect whereas others make them excited. I remember once being in a group with Maxwell Cade, a great pioneer in the study and use of bio-feedback to achieve altered states of consciousness. He talked us through a relaxation session using a spiralling staircase of colour. To my surprise it turned out that some people had exhibited considerable stress while 'imaging' in this way. They found they simply could not picture some of the colours.

Perhaps the funniest example of this kind is the story Max told of a pupil of his who exhibited rising stress levels while taking part in a relaxation session that started with a slow count backwards from ten. Ten, nine, eight, seven, six, five, were bad enough, but four, three, two, one had the man positively quivering with tension. It turned out he was a parachutist and was mentally gearing himself up to leap out of an aeroplane thousands of feet up in the air! Not the best way for him to start a relaxation session.

Obviously you don't need a machine to tell you when you don't enjoy doing something, but it can be fun to test yourself with certain trigger words like 'tumour' or 'cancer' or 'sex' or 'mother-in-law' or 'The Beano-Bag Company' – anything you find emotive. We can then set ourselves to learn *not* to react stressfully at the sound of these words and spare ourselves a great deal of anxiety. Remember the question 'Do you need to change the situation or your reaction to it?'. This is one way of learning how to change your reaction.

Not everyone finds bio-feedbacks helpful. Sometimes people fly into a desperate dither at the very thought of it and find the idea of being 'checked' in this way stressful in itself. This is totally counter-productive and, as with anything else, if it creates more problems than it solves – don't do it. It is perfectly possible to learn to relax without using a machine.

Some of us are so tangled up with stress that we rarely, if ever, relax properly. Some people are not even relaxed when they sleep, they are aware of having clenched their teeth or thrashed about all night, waking unrefreshed in the morning. If we do not know, or have forgotten, how to relax properly then we may need to learn a relaxation technique and start practising it at regular times during the day. The harder this is to do, the more we need to do it.

Different therapists teach different techniques and recommend different amounts of commitment. At Bristol we suggest patients aim for two or three half-hourly sessions a day, but my friend and colleague Ainslie Meares suggested much longer. He liked to see his patients relaxing for hours at a time. Only then, he believed, would they experience a flow-on effect that would help them to stop reacting stressfully throughout the day. He had some impressive results with his methods, but of course he didn't have his patients juicing carrots, visiting healers, doing deep-breathing exercises and so on. He was a man who held that 'only the profound and prolonged reduction of stress can bring about a long-term control of cancer' and consequently he concentrated exclusively on relaxation as therapy.

Although we may need to be reminded of just how to relax properly, it is not all that difficult to relax the body and most people can learn to do this quickly. This is good because physical relaxation is important and helpful, but the skill we most need to acquire is one that relaxes and stills the mind as well as the body. Most people find this much harder to achieve than physical relaxation. In fact the practice of relaxation of the physical body often alerts patients to just how much chatter and fuss is going on in their heads all the time. Learning to control this is the occupation of saints and sages and we shouldn't be too surprised if we find it difficult.

When the goal is to still the mind specifically and not just the body, this is usually referred to as meditation.

Meditation

There are hundreds of books written on meditation techniques and nearly as many specially recorded tapes that offer a background sound of birdsong, waves lapping at the shore, or a voice talking you through, and Bristol is no exception. Some people find tapes helpful to begin with and abandon them later as they develop their own ways of meditating. Some people help themselves create a meditative mood by playing special music, burning sweet-smelling incense, or gazing into a candle. Anything like this is quite acceptable as a means to achieving the goal of inner tranquillity, but it is as well not to rely too heavily on any devices or props. They may not always be available, and in the end we should be able to meditate anywhere, in a bus, on a train, from a hospital bed.

Having just used the phrase 'inner tranquillity' I must hasten to say that I didn't achieve much tranquillity of any sort in the early days of my first meditative endeavours. I was rather unsure of myself and knew that I would feel very embarrassed if anyone discovered me at my efforts. This led to me making my first attempts lying on the floor with my foot braced against the door in case anyone came in. I preferred the prospect of scrambling to my feet with a broken ankle to the thought of trying to explain where meditation fitted into the cancer scene. Naturally this inhibited my progress somewhat, but as the days and weeks passed I gained in confidence. I was really enjoying these sessions and I didn't care who knew it.

I learned early on that 'stilling the mind' is a lot easier said than done. Many people who come to Bristol are disappointed that they spend a good part of each meditation group wondering what they are going to have for supper or trying to decide whether to telephone home tonight. They then jerk back to the realization that they are supposed to be in a state of mindless bliss and so feel the whole thing has been a waste of time. This is far from the case. The goal is not necessarily to get rid of all extraneous thoughts, but eventually we should become detached from them. We observe that there are thoughts intruding into our minds, but the very act of seeing them objectively helps us to detach from them. Gradually we become our own observer. That part of ourselves that is observing is watching, not thinking – there is a part of us that is free from thought. . . .

In just the same way as we can detach ourselves from our thoughts, we can detach ourselves from our worry, our fear, our pain, our suffering. This kind of detachment is the way we begin to release ourselves from the grip these things have on us in our ordinary, waking life. If we practice meditation regularly it offers us more than a small oasis of peace at the beginning and end of the day, its effects flow on and affect times when we are not actually meditating. This is not just good for morale – it's good therapy.

Ainslie Meares had this to say about the value of meditation:

Adrenalin levels are raised by stress and lowered by meditation. In my own experience the hormone levels of some patients with hyperthyroidism have returned to normal after intense meditation . . . in intensive meditation there is a mechanism which can initiate the physiological regression necessary to re-establish the healing process.

He published several books and some incredible case histories in order to show that patients who learn deep relaxation techniques release their own healing potential. (*The Lancet* vol 2, 1981).

I think the effect of stress may be similar to the way Gulliver was tied down by the Lilliputians. Remember those childhood story books with drawings of this giant of a man overpowered by tiny little people who tied him down with hundreds of little stakes and ropes? It was easy to see that no single one of these bits of stick and string could hold the man down, it was the cumulative effect of so many of them that rendered him helpless. Even if we cannot see in our lives anything that in itself could be stressful enough to make us ill, maybe it is the cumulative effect of numerous small things that has finally immobilized our health defences. If during the experience of relaxation and meditation we are released from the hold that even *some* of our stresses have over us, then we may find we are able to shake free of the others.

It is not necessary to discuss and analyse every detail of our lives in order to do this. We have the antidote to our troubles available to us in the silence of our souls.

Unfortunately, experiencing anything approaching inner silence is usually rather a slow process and most people give up too quickly. This is an area surrounded by a lot of popular, but unrealistic goals that herald a quick sense of defeat.

The main difficulty is that the conscious mind gets in the way. The part of ourselves that has been in the front line for most of our lives, plotting, planning, deciding, organizing, worrying and generally reacting to the stimulus of our wordly existence is reluctant to take a back seat. When we enter into a meditative state we are deliberately setting aside the busy conscious mind in favour of a communication with a deeper part of ourselves. It is almost as if the conscious mind resents this, and, in an attempt to keep control, puts up the most awful cacophony of background noise at the first hint at our attempts to achieve another level of consciousness.

The only way to overcome this barrier is through discipline. The conscious mind will play endless games with you in order to stay on top. Naturally if it can stop you even *trying* to step aside from its endless chatter there is no fear of you ever succeeding with your attempts to meditate. So its first trick will probably be to give you a very good and plausible reason for not meditating at all. This is the syndrome in operation when we tell ourselves: 'I'm too tired'; 'This room's too cold'; 'The children will be home soon so it isn't worth it'; 'I'm sure I can meditate while I'm finishing the ironing'; 'I fail to see how lying down trying to think of nothing can affect cancer'.

There isn't one of us who has not argued with ourselves along these lines at some time or another. Even if we manage to resist this subtle manipulation we may not be able to resist the pressure that comes next. If we do set aside the time and attempt to let go of the conscious mind it will most likely kick up the biggest racket ever. It is most demoralizing to put up with this. It is difficult to ignore, harder still to believe that tangling with all this could be doing you the slightest bit of good. The risk now is that we will give up half way through our allotted time, thinking 'What could possibly be the point of that?', 'I knew I wouldn't be any good at this', 'Maybe another technique is the answer, I need a mantra, not this breath-counting method'. Once we start thinking along these lines then the conscious mind has won again.

If we imagine that what we are trying to do in our meditating is to make a connection, like a telephone contact, with a part of ourself that is a long way away, we might know better how to help ourselves achieve this.

Suppose you are caring for a small toddler and while you are playing with this child a very special relative phones you up from the other side of the world. Ideally you would like to say to the child, 'just be quiet and wait a minute while I talk for a little while'. This reasonable request would, more than likely, be greeted with a good deal of resistance. The child likes being the centre of attention and resents you switching your focus to someone else. We are all familiar with the type of performance some children would now indulge in: making more and more noise, demanding attention.

If the child is your conscious mind then the caller is another important part of yourself. This precious part is your inner self, your soul, God, The Collective, your spirit – you can call it what you like. Using this analogy we can see how important it is to discipline the little child. If we break off the telephone connection and return our attention to this noisy little toddler we are teaching it that it can always win our attention in this way. On the other hand, if we persevere with making another contact we are taking a big step forward. One does not need to be a parent to know that this lesson is not going to be learned at one go.

There are bound to be times when we feel that our meditation lacks depth and quality because we are valiantly ignoring the spoiled, indulged performance of our conscious selves, and making a very poor contact with our spirit. This is the equivalent of shouting down the telephone with one finger in your ear while little Johnny drums his heels on the floor in rage. Experiences like this are so unsatisfactory it is small wonder that people give up.

Small wonder either that those organizations, groups and institutions for whom meditation is an essential part of their way of life set rigid and firm rules for their members. Religious orders have regular, established periods during the day for prayer and contemplation. Pupils of the martial arts are set prescribed routines that they must follow. Nobody for whom prayer or meditation is a reality relies on inspiration to get them going and no more should we. Discipline is the way in and the way through.

We were once visited by a man from the north of England, a very practical and successful person who had built up a big business that employed a lot of people. He had a brain tumour and had received all the treatment available to him, and now he wanted to boost his immune system with better nutrition and supplements. He was very reluctant to try meditation. He tried to justify his resistance by giving a logical reason for it, saying things like 'It doesn't work for me' and 'I don't get anything out of it'. When we talked to him it became clear that he had a lot of prejudice about meditation. He associated it with a lot of 'hippy types' and 'layabouts' who smoked illegal substances, wore funny clothes and generally got up to no good. For this reason he had made a couple of half-hearted attempts and then announced that it wasn't worth the trouble.

It was quite obvious to us that he was up against his prejudices here, but he wanted to believe he was making a sensible, unbiased decision. The only way for him to make a judgement about the value of meditation for him was to *experience* it – not think about it or talk about it, but to feel it. He agreed to make an effort to meditate for half an hour twice a day for a month and then come back and talk about it. This time he said it 'wasn't so bad' and by the end of two months he was hooked. Now he was coming back asking for advice about how to handle extraneous thoughts and the barriers being put up by his will. Having overcome, through discipline, the resistance of his intellect, he was now eager to deal with the difficulties created by the spoiled child of his pampered will. More discipline.

We are talking about a loving kind of discipline here. The best way to handle the spoiled child is to ignore him. There is no need to shout or get angry and resentful. Indeed if we do, we invite further reactive behaviour. The same is true for our noisy, intrusive thoughts. We should not fight these, we should ignore them. Indifference and detachment will not give them power; anger and disappointment most certainly will.

A tip from one of our counsellors for those times when the conscious mind is being particularly disruptive: go for a walk. She has found that a short, steadying walk round the block or in the garden is a way of using movement to disperse surface tension, and this seems to calm everything down a bit.

Patients sometimes come back to the Centre saying they are disgusted and annoyed with themselves because they are such a hopeless failure when it comes to meditation. The longer they go on reacting in this way, the longer they will put off that wonderful day when the background noise dies down. The toddler looks up with a sigh and a shrug when the telephone rings and withdraws into his own world until you have finished talking. Yes, it really does happen, and it is worth waiting for.

Practical Techniques

The preparation for relaxation and meditation is the same.

Most people only know two states of being: awake and asleep. Sometimes even that is not too clear. When they are meant to be awake they are half asleep, and when they are in bed asleep their minds are restless and buzzing. In relaxation you are awake and aware, but relaxed and peaceful at the same time. You are not going to lose consciousness and go into a trance. You are quite safe.

If you can, choose a special place for your relaxation sessions. Somewhere in your home that you particularly like that you can make your special corner. This isn't essential (I haven't a square yard in my home that I could call my own), but I think it helps if you can create a little bit of atmosphere to come back to each time. If you are working it might be easier to get out of the office at midday and do your relaxation in a park nearby, alternating with the local church or library in the winter.

If you are reading this from a hospital ward you have very little choice about where to work from. Don't worry about it, you can relax any time, anywhere, I'm only trying to make it easier. Again, don't worry if you have to do this exercise in bed, but if possible choose somewhere else. The problem with bed is that we associate it with sleep, and when you first start learning to relax there is a great temptation to go to sleep, and this is not the object of the exercise. If possible do this exercise in a firm armchair, something not too squishy.

If you are in pain, or for any reason find it uncomfortable to do this sitting upright, then adjust your position. You can lie down flat if you prefer or prop yourself up with pillows and cushions. As far as possible, keep your spine straight.

1. Push your bottom well to the back of the chair and sit up comfortably straight with your back supported by the chair.

2. Take off spectacles and loosen your clothing – neck-ties and belts.
3. Check that your neck is straight, that your chin is not dropping on your chest or stuck up in the air.
4. Arrange your hands and arms so that they are not clutching at anything or helping to support you. Check that your shoulders are not hunched.
5. Mentally scan your body for tension and discomfort. This is the time to have a little wriggle, scratch your nose, clear your throat. If you notice tension in a particular part of your body, tighten the muscles around that area and then release. You will relax your jaw considerably if you open your mouth wide and stick your tongue out for a moment or two. Some people like to tense and then relax different muscles systematically throughout the body; for others this is not necessary. Do what feels right for you.
6. Once you feel comfortable imagine the force of gravity taking over and sense yourself sinking into the chair. Feel the chair, or whatever is supporting you, taking your weight. Feel it holding you. Let yourself sink deeper and deeper.
7. Give yourself permission to withdraw your interest and attention from the things that are going on around you. You can still hear and sense the outside world, but you are withdrawing from those things.
8. Allow yourself to focus your attention on your breathing. Feel the breath cooling your nostrils and passing into your chest. Let your abdomen rise slightly to accommodate the filling lungs. In a few moments your breathing will become steadier.
9. Gradually your breathing will slow down. You may notice that you breathe in and then out and then experience a little pause after the outbreath. This pause may get longer as your breathing gets slower. Allow your lungs to take in and expel breath in their own time.

10. Continue breathing in this way, checking from time to time that your body has not tensed up without you knowing it. Have you started frowning? Are you clenching your jaw? Or gripping with your hands? If so, just let go again of those parts of you, feel them relaxing, and breathe the tension out on your next exhalation.

This state of unstressed awareness is what we mean by relaxation. This is the moment to vary your relaxation according to temperament and need.

If your aim is to meditate you need do nothing more than what you are doing already but add to the relaxation of your physical body your intention to relax the activity of your mind as well. Some of the oldest meditation traditions suggest doing this by focusing attention on the breath. Slow mental counting: one, two, three, four on the in breath – pause – one, two, three, four on the out breath, acts as a distraction from your thoughts. Another way would be to count more slowly, counting each in and out breath as one, going up to four, and then starting again. In either case you are reminding yourself to focus your attention on your breathing, not on the clatter that may be going on around you.

During the course of meditation you may realize that you have just returned to an awareness of your breath, but you have been away somewhere else for a while. You may not know quite what has happened to you: you were not asleep, you were not daydreaming – you were there, but you were not there. This is a sweetly exquisite experience that is beyond words. If it happens to you, you will know for yourself why people make such a song and dance about meditation and you will never have to make yourself do it ever again. You will never want to stop.

If you feel you are not ready to transcend thought through merely focusing on or counting the breath, when you have reached a state of slow relaxed breathing you could offer your mind something peaceful to do.

1. Imagine something positive and wonderful that you would like to have: joy, peace, healing, strength, forgiveness – anything you like – and literally breathe it in with each breath. This can be called **virtue breathing**. Now allow yourself to exhale a negative, opposite feeling. Imagine sorrow, pain, sickness, helplessness and guilt flowing out of you and away. Settle for two things that have meaning for you personally and breathe them in and out until you want to work with something else, then change. Try inhaling peace and exhaling fear for a minute or two, then see what comes to mind.

2. An alternative to this would be to make a slow positive affirmation in harmony with your gentle rhythmic breathing. Something like 'all is well, there is nothing to fear' or 'my body is healing itself now' would be simple and easy.

3. You could finish your relaxation with some deeper breathing, intended to oxygenate the body. Read more about this in the section on breathing.

Use whatever aids you like. Special rugs or cushions to sit on, sweet-smelling flowers or joss sticks in the room, or music playing quietly in the background, may help to distract you from the background noise that often hinders progress at the beginning. Eventually you may be able to manage without any of these things.

Both India and the yoga tradition, and China and the Taoist movement believe that correct breathing is the way to enlightenment and healthy living.

If you do decide to pursue meditation seriously you could experiment with your physical position. Gradually introduce yourself to feeling less comfortable when you begin. As you then continue to achieve deep levels of relaxation you will have the satisfaction of knowing that it is your mind that is relaxing your body and not the other way around. This is a considerable achievement, and is likely to take a lot of practice, so I do not advise tangling with the Full Lotus on day one. An excellent position to try would be kneeling with your buttocks on your heels. Chuang Tzu, an early philosopher of the Tao, declared that the perfect man 'breathes through his heels' and this is assumed to be a reference to this posture. He talks about meditative breathing as 'the fasting mind . . .'

One of the oldest Chinese medical classics, the *Ling-shu*, has an entire chapter devoted to breathing. It recommends visualizing the breath tracking the path of two meridians. One that runs up the spine, over the head, bisecting the forehead and nose, and connecting with another that flows up from the genitals, through the navel, the sternum and the chin. This pathway covers breathing centres characteristically used in Tantric yoga, and to imagine the breath circulating around the body along these channels can be immensely powerful. This is discussed in a most informative and poetical way by Chang Chung-yuan in his book *Creativity and Taoism*. This is a book that goes into great detail, but may be worth dipping into for inspiration.

Useful names and addresses

The British Wheel of Yoga
Grafton Grange
Grafton
York

Audio Limited
26–28 Wendell Road
London W12
Contact Audio Limited if you are interested in bio-feedback as an aid to meditation. They are a source of machines and run courses in how to use them.

Information about autogenic training and therapy from
British Association for Autogenic Training
101 Harley Street
London W1

Breathing

'I will cause breath to enter you, and ye shall live' *Ezekiel 37, 5*

If you are one of those people that prefer to start with the physical benefits of therapy it may help you to think of your breathing exercises as a way of oxygenating the body.

Air is an essential element for man. It is true that we need to be nourished through regular food intake and maintain our high percentage of water through frequent drinking, but we can actually survive long periods without food and water. I have known people who have lived without food for weeks, and there are many known cases of people surviving quite long periods without water, but without breath most of us would be dead in minutes. The only exception to this seems to be cases of people drowning in very cold water, and later being revived successfully. However this would be exceptional.

Recent years have seen us finally sit up and take notice of what we are putting in our mouths, maybe good breathing will be the next health craze. I wouldn't be surprised.

Like everything else, of course, it won't be new, just a revival of the old. The best breathing exercises are taught in classes for ancient martial arts training and yoga practice, both centuries old. Again, as with so many things, we have to unlearn first. Even if we didn't go to the kind of school that taught 'chins up and chests out' and twice round the tennis courts with a book on our heads (yes, you've guessed, that was me) it is likely we have a sort of parade-ground attitude to breathing.

Most people think deep breathing consists of lifting your shoulders up to your ears and thrusting your chest forward. Unfortunately this kind of vigorous over-breathing does us very little good, in fact, quite the reverse. It leads to hyperventilation, a condition that is currently being held responsible for a great many minor ills and ailments. I admit it makes a refreshing change from blaming everything on 'allergies', and it is a lot easier to treat. Poor breathing techniques that lead to hyperventilation result in a deficiency of carbon dioxide which can be redressed by the simple expedient of putting your head in a brown paper bag and breathing in more carbon dioxide. It is truly amazing what you can do to yourself by altering your breathing techniques. I know all about hyperventilation because it was the only guaranteed way of making yourself faint at the feet of the hockey coach and get yourself off school games.

The idea of effecting a cure for anything by putting your head in a large, brown paper bag is so charmingly eccentric I should be sorry to see it pass into history, but it would be better from every point of view if we learned to control our breathing in a more constructive way.

Breathing exercises are part of the Bristol Programme.

Why? Why does breathing matter?

In all the major religious traditions breath is associated with a very special life force. It is variously known as 'spirit' or 'prana' or 'chi' but behind the semantics is a shared belief that man can empower himself through conscious, directed breathing. In addition to this, the cancer patient may benefit from the resulting improvement in oxygen uptake.

One of the very many fascinating things I learned about cancer from Josef Issels was that cancer cells don't need oxygen in order to survive. They thrive in starvation conditions and actually do not like the presence of oxygen. Working from this premise Issels had incorporated into his therapy two specific treatments designed to oxygenate the body. One of these involved injecting huge syringes filled with ozone into the biggest muscles he could find. This was horribly painful but appeared to be perfectly safe. The other method involved extracting some of your blood, oxygenating it and putting it back. The only trouble with this was that what went back contained sizeable bubbles. I used to watch, terrified, as this was slowly returned to my pulsing veins, wondering whether it would be easier to die from a stroke than from cancer. I think, on balance, it is kinder not to have to mull over such choices. Anyway these methods are not available in this country – certainly not to someone trying to help themselves. Dr Bruce Halstead at his clinic in California uses a method involving a decompression chamber, but I have not heard of this being done anywhere else.

It is true to say that there are experts who do not share Issels' views concerning oxygenation. I have been told by physicists working in this field that it is impossible to get oxygen to the site of the cancer in anything but paltry quantities. The blood supplies to tumours are usually scanty and inadequate and oxygen would have to be pumped at pressures that would be quite unacceptable. We are in much the same position here as with many other self-help remedies. There are factors that point towards oxygenation being helpful, but disagreement as to how helpful, and doubts about the practicalities of treatment. The decision to pursue oxygen therapy in spite of this is based on two factors. One is that good breathing and better oxygenation are positive health factors in a general over-all sense even if little direct impact is made on the cancer cells. The second reason that makes this idea very appealing is that it is so simple to learn oxygenation techniques and costs us nothing except a few minutes of our time.

1. Find somewhere warm and comfortable where you can lie down.
2. Consciously relax your body by mentally checking out where the tensions are and letting go.
3. Bring your attention to your breathing and concentrate on it. Allow yourself to do this for as long as it takes for your breathing to slow down, and for a slight pause to develop between the out breath and the in breath.
4. Now put your hands over your abdomen, fingers touching loosely just above your navel. Feel your fingers moving up and slightly apart as you breathe in. Experience this for a while.

5. Next move your hands upwards and apart and place them at the side of your body. Here you will feel them being gently pushed outwards as your lungs expand. Experience this for a while.
6. Finally put one of your hands on your sternum, under your throat, and feel the movement there too.
7. Now put your hands back on the floor, lying loosely at your sides. Think of your lungs filling up from the bottom. Remember that slight push on your diaphragm that caused your tummy to rise up a little. Remember the gentle sideways expansion of your ribs and the soft rise and fall of your chest. Imagine every part of your lungs filling with air and passing oxygen into your blood. Imagine your blood washing it over every cell in your body. Imagine the cancer cells dying because of these changed conditions.

Repeat this exercise several times a day. It is easy to do this at the beginning or end of a meditation, relaxation or visualization session. Of course you can do it standing up, either at an open window or on a country walk, but if you do, make sure that you think of breathing from the bottom half of your lungs first and avoid hunching your shoulders.

Another way of oxygenating the blood would be by aerobic exercise. The thought of this may fill you with alarm, and of course you should not attempt any such thing if your idea of exercise before you got cancer was lifting a pint of beer to your lips. But if you are physically fit – and many cancer patients are – then don't rule out this possibility. Talk it over with your doctor if you are in any doubt and then think about how you are going to do it. Aerobic exercise should not be violent and you should work your way into it slowly. Don't fling yourself on to the streets trying to run a mile if you don't even walk to the shops. Start by walking, progress to walking at a brisk pace, graduate to jogging if you feel like it.

The story of Belinda Carlton, told in her book *Big is Invisible* is an inspiring tale. In 1982 she was recovering from a series of operations for cancer and weighed over twenty stone. In 1984 she completed the London marathon in 4 hours 25 minutes. Her son-in-law acted as her trainer and her instructions for her first week were:

> Monday: go for a walk; Tuesday: walk briskly for five minutes; Wednesday: walk slowly for ten minutes; Thursday: walk for fifteen minutes, stop if necessary; Friday: rest; Saturday: walk for five minutes.

Another obvious way to exercise would be to join an aerobics class and be guided through exercises that are specially designed to oxygenate the body. Some of these classes can be rather violent so remember to join a *beginners'* class, and be prepared to go at your own pace. If you can't face the thought of this, don't worry. Any activity performed steadily for about 15 to 20 minutes that makes you pink and warm all over is aerobic. Take note: this is not likely to be golf. Sorry about that. It could be, but only if you set out with that intention. It could be cycling, jogging or swimming, though, and these are all fairly cheaply and readily available.

Remember not to strain yourself. If you perform your chosen activity for a longer time you need not work hard in order to achieve impressive results. I discovered this at our local swimming bath. I took myself along there to try a little gentle movement to strengthen my muscles after a lumpectomy operation. Wondering what percentage of a mile my modest few lengths might have scored, I foolishly enquired of the young, track-suited Adonis at the edge of the pool how many lengths there are in a mile. He looked down with pity and asked condescendingly, 'Why do you want to know?' Before I could stop myself I said, 'Because I was thinking of doing one.'

Sixty four.

Of course I had to do it. It practically took all day, but I had to do it. I was actually able to walk back to the changing rooms unaided, but it was touch and go. The interesting part was that

I felt wonderful. My legs felt a bit wobbly because of the unaccustomed exercise, but I was aglow. I was tingling all over and I felt energized in every pore of my body. I even got a certificate and a badge to sew on my costume. Much more to the point I got the swimming bug. I never push myself. I often swim a mile but at a slow, leisurely pace. I settle to an uncompetitive speed that feels comfortable. There is no strain at all, but if I keep going long enough I feel that glow creeping over me and I know I am oxygenating every corner of myself and it feels great.

If anyone had suggested to me that I should swim so much as a hundred yards when I was first ill I would not have been too pleased. There is a time and a place for everything, but be open to the idea that you might, like Belinda Carlton, be capable of more than you think.

Coping with emotions

Although I do think it is sensible to get some professional help in this area whenever possible, there are bound to be circumstances when you can't. In that case you can do a great deal to help yourself. Women often find it easier to admit that they have emotional problems than men, but men might be interested to hear what John Cleese has to say about his experience:

> Men particularly tend to hold in their emotions. Men are much madder than women. At an age when women are learning something about their emotions, men are learning Bradman's batting averages off by heart.

Emotional stress is often created and aggravated by the fact that we do not express our emotions properly. There may be quite a lot of denial going on, which means that much of what we feel may be suppressed. Naturally our personalities have been party to this suppression and so we should be as objective and detached as possible when engaging in exercises to do with emotional expression. Before you start it would be a good idea to do the exercise described at the beginning of the chapter 'How to Start Helping Yourself' (page 167). In doing this you will be better able to work from the perspective of that part of you that is detached from your immediate experiences. This is sometimes referred to as getting in touch with your own 'Wise Observer'. This is the part of you that is not tangled up with feelings and emotions and is able to think clearly.

Another 'disengaging' exercise would be to relax comfortably in a quiet place and say to yourself:

'I have a body, but I am not my body.'
'I have a mind full of thoughts and opinions, but I am not my thoughts and opinions.'
'I have feelings and emotions, but I am not my feelings and emotions.'

This helps you to become aware that you have an existence that is not ruled by your body, your mind or your emotions. You need to understand this if you are going to be your own counsellor.

Much of the purpose of counselling is to help us face up to aspects of ourselves that we have been avoiding throughout life. We can do this for ourselves if we start by accepting that we only perform in the world with one facet of ourselves. There are quite a few more actors and actresses backstage trying to make themselves heard and play their part, but we are trying to ignore them. We ignore them because we have been taught to favour certain ways of expressing ourselves and suppress others. Try to imagine yourself as a whole family of people, not just the one everybody thinks you are. Even the most brave and confident types have a nervous, timid person inside them. Here are a few stereotypes for you to think about.

The Fearful Baby
The Playful Child
The Daring Optimist

The Gloomy Pessimist
The Home-maker
The Explorer
The Frivolous Hedonist
The Wise Philosopher
The Loving Parent
The Impeccable Warrior

John Cleese has talked about the struggle he has between his Managing Director and his Chairman, both of whom have very definite ideas about how he should lead his life. You could add those to the list.

Imagine yourself as all of these people. Play around with this list. Add to it and fill out the details. If you are married, with children and have a cosy home then your Home-maker and your Loving Parent parts of your personality have had a chance to express themselves. But if you have achieved this at the expense of your career and feel trapped in your domestic life, then your Explorer and Wise Philosopher might be having a thin time of it.

Very few of us live harmoniously with all the different aspects of ourselves. We are usually busy denying or smothering something. Accepting that there may be facets of ourselves that we have lost touch with may present something of a challenge. The challenging part is admitting that we are capable of behaving in lots of different ways, and maybe, as a result of this, we shall find conflict within ourselves. If we are a whole family of personalities and not just the one we show to the world, we must get to know this family better, and harmonize our internal relationships.

This does require a certain amount of skill and cunning since some of our sub-personalities (which is how we can refer to these different parts of ourselves) are in conflict with each other. It would be tricky for example to be a Playful Child and an Impeccable Warrior at the same time, but it is a mistake to imagine the same person cannot express herself in these ways at different times. Elderly, childless people are going to wonder how they are ever going to express the role of loving parent. Perhaps they will never experience this role in a literal sense, but they can apply it in their relationship to the younger generation as a whole and know how it feels. Our ability to behave in many different ways and not get stuck with one performance has a lot to do with our emotions.

Our emotions represent ways of responding to our experiences in life. Despite the Great British Public School tradition, which would have us believe otherwise, God in all His wisdom created us with the capacity to respond with feeling to the world. *The appropriate expression of emotion is a way of discharging the potentially stressful effect that deep feelings can have on us.* Read that sentence again, it's important.

Suppressed emotions can cause us a lot of physical as well as mental problems. Emotions that are driven down inside us and not expressed can create a build-up of stress in the body. This leads to tension and myriad physical ailments from backache to migraine. Possibly even to cancer.

Most of us do not express our emotions appropriately. We have been taught and trained not to. If small boys are punished and mocked for crying, they will soon learn to stop. In our culture Big Boys Don't Cry – or at least they didn't when I was a girl, with the result that I see hundreds of men of my generation who haven't cried for thirty or forty years. Girls, on the other hand, were allowed to cry, but they weren't allowed to get angry. Consequently I meet a lot of women who cry all the time, and not only when they are sad.

Two things are important. One is that emotions should be expressed. The word itself – e-motion – means 'movement away from'. Secondly they should be expressed appropriately.

Sometimes people who would describe themselves as 'emotional' are not actually expressing themselves appropriately. What often happens is that we attach ourselves to one particular emotional response – probably encouraged by school and family – and we stick with this one at the expense of others. Women who cry are often like this. I often hear from women that they have been very angry about something, but when I ask what they did about it they say, 'I burst into tears, of course'. This is not an appropriate use of tears.

Look for a moment at the five basic categories of emotional response:

Anger/shouting
Fear/groaning
Grief/weeping
Sympathy/humming
Love/laughing.

I have linked each emotion with a sound or form of expression. I have drawn these from various sources to make a simple useful model to work with. Which ones are you happy about and which ones make you feel uncomfortable? Can you see one that you favour most? Is there one that you consciously avoid? If this is true you are likely to be using your emotions inappropriately. This will mean that half the time your emotional outpourings will only serve to puzzle and annoy the people around you and not help you very much.

If we are to use our emotions in order to release some of the tension and stress that has built up in us over the years, two conditions must prevail. We must be *allowed* to do so and we must feel that it is *safe*. If you have a history of being denied emotional outlets, then permission is particularly important. You must give yourself permission. It may help to know that I give you permission and all the staff at Bristol give you permission, because if you were with us we would all be encouraging you to do this. Now give yourself permission. You may find this easier to do if you see yourself as your own 'loving parent'. To feel safe you will have to choose your own time and place.

I hit on this business of giving myself permission quite accidentally. I was in Germany about a month after having the cancer diagnosed. I was still full of fear and shock; I was dreadfully homesick; I was mourning my dead parents, who I now missed more than ever; and I had been trying not to cry for weeks on end. My fierce admonitions to myself that I must not cry because once I started I would never stop had not been very successful. I was never far from tears. I never had a good cry, but my eyes pricked all the time and I felt dreadful. One day I could stand it no longer. I set aside an entire afternoon and a jumbo box of tissues and settled down for a good cry. I deliberately thought about all the things that were making me sad and allowed myself to weep about them. After a few minutes I dried up, so I pressed all the buttons again, and had another little go. After a few more minutes I dried up again. This time when I ran through the saga of my sorrows, nothing happened at all. I quite simply could not believe it. I had the whole afternoon stretching ahead of me and I had run out of tears. I learned some very important things that day.

If you allow yourself an emotional outlet for your feelings you will gain control over them, not lose it. Unexpressed emotions make a great deal of fuss and bother in the background, so much so that we fear them and suppress them more. This creates a vicious circle in which we convince ourselves that any expression of these feelings would result in uncontrollable drama. In fact the reverse is true. If our emotions are acknowledged and expressed they quieten down. There is no need for them to haunt us if they know they have their rightful place. There is no need for them to hurt other people either, and this is what often lurks at the back of our minds when we think about being angry.

Anger

In my experience anger is the emotion least understood and most feared. I meet a lot of people who say they have never, ever, lost their tempers. But if I ask their family what they are like to live with I do not necessarily hear that these people are equable and patient. Far from it. Not losing your temper does not mean you never feel angry. This anger has to go somewhere and if it is not harmlessly discharged, or put to good use, it will be bottled up. Often people who never lose their tempers are resentful, moody types who bear grudges and sulk. At the end of the day this kind of behaviour is a lot harder to live with.

One of my favourite patients at Bristol was a man of over seventy who said he had been a Boy Scout in his youth and Baden-Powell in person had addressed his troop one day. Apparently he said to them, 'Keep your temper, boys, nobody else wants it'! This is a very succinct example of the misconception that it is dangerous to discharge emotions. There are safe ways of doing this. It is more dangerous *not* to.

Anger is so often associated with violence: we are afraid we shall do physical damage to another, or be hurt ourselves. This is less likely to be the case if we explode with a roar of 'You can't be serious!' than if we rumble along with resentment. In the first case the anger is being expressed harmlessly and to the person concerned, in the latter it festers away unexpressed and may well coming flying to the surface later in the presence of an otherwise innocent observer who just has the bad luck to trigger it off. This uncontrolled anger of the 'kick the cat' variety is what everyone is afraid of because it is destructive. But anger has a constructive, purposeful function too.

It is our way of saying 'no' to the world. It is part of our self-defence. It identifies our boundaries. Not only this, if we acknowledge that we are angry, we are saying to ourselves 'I don't want this' and this is the first step towards changing it. Anger should motivate us to take action. It is rare for me to meet patients who reacted angrily to the news that they had cancer, but when I do I know they will have the most terrific motivation for self-help.

It is possible to exercise control over anger, but only if you acknowledge your angry feelings when you get them, and promise yourself that you will allow yourself to express this feeling. Maybe not at the time, but later. You can now sit seething in front of your boss at a committee meeting and tell yourself that you will allow yourself to express this anger later. As long as you are faithful to that promise you will find you become less vulnerable to the tension and frustration that some of our life experiences bring. After all, nobody wants to scream and carry on during the meeting, toss all the papers into the air, storm out and slam the door off its hinges. (Although I think we have a sneaking affection on occasions for people who do. Remember Nikita Khruschev taking off his shoe at the United Nations and banging it on the table?) The fact that we may prefer not to express our feelings *any*where at *any*time makes it all the more important to make a pact with ourselves that we shall express them *some*where at *some*time. As soon as we do this we take control of the situation.

Find a quiet corner and allow yourself to rant and rage. If you have literally never lost your temper you may never have shouted either. Just see what you can do. You may have to start small and work up. I made my first attempts at expressing anger by saying 'bugger' in a miserable little whisper, only getting it into a full-bloodied roar after lots of practice. Naturally this is not the sort of thing to do in a crowded restuarant. In fact the more space you have the better. I share with one of my colleagues who works with emotional discharge, the view that emotions should be expressed through sound and movement. Remember the time when you were small and you used to stamp your feet when you were cross, and start shouting? (No doubt you also remember your mother saying 'Don't you raise your voice at me' but we'll gloss over that.) Stamping is a good idea, but if you end up doing this exercise in your car in a remote lay-by stamping would be difficult. You might ball a fist and thump the steering wheel instead. Once you have allowed yourself to do this you'll find a way.

Now apply these principles to other emotions.

Fear

This is another of the so-called 'negative' emotions that we all feel we should have grown out of. Just because we are no longer afraid of the dark we tell ourselves there isn't anything else to be afraid of. Not true. We need to know what fear is. This most primitive of feelings is the one that alerts us to danger. Without it we would never survive. Like anger, it motivates us for action and tells us when to make important changes in our lives. If we are not aware of this signal that our mind gives us when we are at risk, then we are vulnerable indeed and will not live long.

It is an unusual patient who does not react fearfully to the news that they have cancer. Equally it would be an unusual person who felt they wanted to groan with fear at the time they were given the news. In a hospital ward with a circle of strangers at the end of the bed is not the ideal moment. I think choosing the appropriate time for the expression of emotion is especially important with fear. This may be linked to its connection with survival in our more primitive past, when it may have been important not to show you were afraid. This might have given us a tactical advantage then, and it is possible we are reacting in much the same way now when we grit our teeth in the determination not to let anyone know how scared we are. But if we are scared then that feeling has to go somewhere, and if we drive it deep down inside us it will cause stress and hinder our progress to good health. Like anger it can be safely discharged in a controlled way, in our own time, when we feel safe.

Grief

When I cried in Germany I was weeping from a great sense of loss. I was cut off from my husband and children, I was lonely, I had lost my health and, as far as I could see, my future. Crying was my way of allowing myself to feel all this.

While it is true that most people are more tolerant and less afraid of tears than they are of anger and fear, it is not always easy to cry in the presence of others. This too may have to be a very private moment. Watch out here for the people who tell you you ought to have a good cry and then more or less prescribe how long you are allowed. They accompany their assistance with remarks like 'Come on now, that's enough' or 'John will be home in a minute, you don't want him to see you like this, do you?' Try to see the funny side of this and mentally make arrangements to do a proper job for yourself later on. Some people are actually quite entertaining in the way they react to tears, leaping about looking for tissues or handkerchiefs with which they literally try to push the tears back into you.

Try if you can to make sure that you are using tears to express grief. You may have a Spoiled Child in you who has indulged herself with weeping as a way of expressing orgies of self-pity. This kind of performance will not result in healthy discharge. Only your Wise Observer will be able to tell you if you have developed bad habits. A common trick of the Spoiled Child would be to use tears in order to get its own way. Tearful manipulation of this sort is self-indulgent, not therapeutic. Ask yourself directly, 'Do I have a need to release my feelings through tears?'

Finally, it may be important in the case of weeping that we should eventually be able to cry in the presence of others. Some therapists believe that 'permission to cry in public' may be an important breakthrough.

Sympathy

Sympathy and understanding are feelings that pave the way for love. If we sense that people are aware of us, know what our problems are, we can begin to trust them, to feel open to them. Only then, when we feel we are safe with them, can we allow them to love us, or believe that they will love us. Interestingly enough, people who are good at giving sympathy and understanding are often not good at receiving it. This may link in with the fact that many people take up 'caring' work (where sympathy becomes a profession) because they have a low self-image and need to justify themselves with good deeds all the time. This was certainly true of me. I was very hot on sympathy, but I never felt I was getting the understanding I wanted from others. It came as quite a surprise to listen to an old friend of mine telling me I was difficult to reach. If you feel you are not getting enough sympathy or understanding it may be that you need to work on the idea that you are entitled to it, and the world will not reel backwards with shock if you ask for it.

If you find it difficult to be sympathetic towards others the situation is slightly different. More than likely you see sympathy as an indulgence. You are afraid that if you show the smallest degree of understanding you will be swamped and there will be no end to it all. If there is someone close to you who is extremely demanding and always looking for an opening in the conversation to start telling you their troubles, you may cut them off by withholding your interest. Actually if you could just attend to them for a while with a few well-placed 'Mmms' and 'Hmms' you will find that by meeting their need in this way you have saved yourself a lot of trouble as well. They will no longer need to keep asking you for attention. They will have gained the reassurance they needed and you will have opened up in a way that is very important. This is a two-way process. If you can't give understanding, you can't receive it. This is the meaning of the word 'compassion': it means entering and sharing an experience.

If you can't sympathize, you can't love. If you think you are loving someone without understanding them, then as like as not you are only bargaining: 'I love you like this, but not like that'. We all know that love of this kind is hardly worth having. We want to be known for what we are, accepted and understood, and then loved. By learning to give and take sympathy and understanding we are opening ourselves to the possibility of unconditional love.

Love

Love and laughter are expressions of happiness and warmth, feelings that we are often moved to express through touch. Unfortunately we have slid into the habit of making less and less physical contact with each other in a casual, friendly sort of way. In fact we often apologize if we accidentally touch someone's hand, and snatch our own away quickly. More and more the loving touch has come to be associated with sexual activity. This has loaded everything with tension and meaning and led to a sad diminution of a vital part of our expression as loving people.

Children who are not cuddled and caressed do not thrive. Underweight babies receiving hospital care are given TLC (tender loving care) as part of their treatment, because everyone knows that this will encourage them to grow and flourish. Chimpanzee babies, deprived of the touch of their own kind, will simply die for the need of it.

The kind of laughter that bubbles up in us as an expression of well-being and contentment is itself a healing force, as Norman Cousins has described in his book, *Anatomy of an Illness*. Nobody is yet quite sure why laughter should have a therapeutic effect, but it is possible that it stimulates the release of a special endorphin into the blood. Tests done at the Vienna Neurological Clinic showed that blood serum from people hypnotized into a happy, cheerful state dealt more rapidly with typhoid baccilli than blood from people hypnotized into a sad, depressed frame of mind.

Most of us are hungry for love and will have experienced times in our lives when we had to compete for it and there never seemed to be enough. And in some ways that is true, there is not a lot of it about. Certainly unconditional love, though much talked of, is a bit thin on the ground. This is because our potential for love is harnessed by fear. Read Jampolski's beautiful book, *Love is Letting Go of Fear* (see Suggested reading, page 131). If we are open to the giving and receiving of love we are becoming part of the most powerful force in the universe. The Chinese refer to Love as 'The Great Controller', acknowledging that ultimately all our emotions are subject to this one.

Even when our human efforts look a bit weedy we know that God is Love and that He loves us unconditionally. We can lean into His love endlessly and know that it is limitless and endless. As we learn more and more about love we will find that it is actually possible to handle everything that comes our way with love.

Gradually we shall have less need to respond with anger, fear, grief or sympathy because, by understanding these emotions better we shall gain control over them. Once we have achieved this we can choose to detach from these responses and use only love. When we do this we start 'seeing from the heart'.

It is only with the heart that one can see rightly; what is essential is invisible to the eye.
'What is essential is invisible to the eye,' the little prince repeated, so that he would be sure to remember.
The Little Prince by Antoine de St Exupéry.

Combine this work on your emotions with the use of Bach Flower Remedies, pages 185–190.

Summary

* Emotions can and should be expressed. Their suppression can cause dangerous internal stress.
* They *can* be expressed safely – even negative ones.
* In this way you will *gain* control over them, not lose it.

*   You must allow yourself to express emotion, give yourself permission.

*   You should continue expressing your emotion until it feels right to stop.

*   Whenever possible emotions should be expressed through sound and action.

Suggested reading
How to Meditate by Lawrence Le Shan
You Can Fight For Your Life by Lawrence Le Shan (Thorsons)
The Wealth Within by Ainslie Meares (Ashgrove Press)
The Cloud of Unknowing Author not known (Penguin)
Silent Music by William Johnson (Collins)
Love is Letting Go of Fear by Gerald Jampolski (Celestial Arts, California)

I THINK THEREFORE I AM

GLENDOWER   I can call spirits from the vasty deep.
HOTSPUR   Why, so can I, or so can any man;
             But will they come when you do call for them?
                        Henry IV, Part 1, Act III, scene 1

I think most of us are aware that we have more powers than we use. We sense that man has a quality and a capacity that he has lost touch with. We watch television pictures of yogis in India lying down in the road and being rolled over by American trucks and then getting up, dusting themselves off, and walking away to an accompanying clatter of camera shutters. We ask ourselves what on earth is going on here. What does the man *do* that enables his body to withstand such an insult? Could we do it? Are we afraid that Hotspur might be right — that it won't work if *we* try it?

Most of us will go so far as to admit that mind can exercise the most powerful influence over matter, but we doubt whether we ourselves could ever do anything so spectacular. No need to be too ambitious. We don't want to summon spirits from the vasty deep, nor feel the tread of an American truck, but it would be nice to improve our healing capacity. Evidence suggests that we can.

We know that physical performance is influenced by mental processes but as yet we do not fully understand this connection. Children in Japan who are allergic to poison ivy have been tested, perhaps rather heartlessly, to establish how much influence their own expectations have on their auto-immune reaction (Y. Ikemi and S. Nakagawa; *Kyushi Journal of Medical Science*, vol 13, 1962). The results have been quite dramatic. If the children are blindfolded and informed that their arms are to be brushed by poison ivy they react violently with symptoms of swelling, erythema and itching. They will do this even if they are in fact being touched by something quite harmless like grass, provided that they *believe* it to be poison ivy. Fascinating to report, the reverse is also true: if they are told that the poison ivy is grass, then nothing happens at all. In other words, these children can induce and suppress symptoms according to their expectations.

Denial

In recent months I have had many letters in response to a television interview. Without a doubt the most interesting of these was from a woman who told me about her experience with Hodgkin's disease. During her stay in hospital it became clear very quickly that her situation was serious, but she insisted that she did not want to be told any bad news. She agreed to cooperate in every way with the doctors, but refused to be party to any discussions. If there was anything to be said, they could say it to her husband. She then proceeded to undergo chemotherapy treatment which she told me she 'enjoyed', a response which, in my experience of patient feedback, I would say was quite unique. Her husband on the other hand, had a very miserable time of it. He suffered the typical side-effects of her treatment of nausea and vomiting, and after a few weeks his hair started falling out. Meanwhile the patient herself sailed on cheerfully, 'thoroughly enjoying' the time spent in hospital. When it was finally revealed to her that she had had cancer she reacted angrily, saying, if it was that serious she should have been told in the first place. I venture to suggest that she was wrong.

This lady's case exhibits clearly some interesting facets of the healing process. First, she was practising 'denial'. We know from the work done at King's College Hospital in a trial conducted with breast cancer patients that survival seems to be affected by the patients' attitude. And the same might be true of all cancer patients. The woman who wrote to me dogmatically refused to hear how ill she was, would not take part in any discussions about treatment, and therefore had no fears or negative expectations concerning the chemotherapy. None of these things was true for her husband. Not only did he take on all the negative programming on her behalf and respond accordingly, he was cast in the role of scapegoat as well. Anthropological observations of societies where magic and medicine work hand in hand tell us that disease is often dealt with in this way. Men groan outside the hut while women give birth inside. Even the modern twentieth-century man who charms warts may use an outside agent for dispersal – hopefully not human.

I do not believe that it is necessary for anyone to take on the suffering or the side-effects for denial to be effective, but this is a most interesting story.

Denial of this sort is a hard act to follow. Personally I was quite incapable of such a performance, but I have met others who do much the same. We had a patient at the Centre once who said there had been nothing really wrong with her breast, but the surgeon had removed it 'just to be on the safe side'. In all fairness to both parties, I find this hard to believe. But all credit to the woman for insisting that the surgeon go along with her refusal to believe that anything serious was happening to her, and all credit to him for realizing this was what she wanted and supporting her in it. What fascinated me about this particular lady was that she came to the Bristol Centre at all. Perhaps at some non-verbal level she was not denying the seriousness of her situation, who knows. Generally speaking, people who can successfully practise denial have no need for a Centre like ours.

Active and positive visualization is a form of denial. When we tell our bodies they are *not* going to deteriorate, suffer pain, experience nausea or any other physical side-effect, we are, in a sense, denying that we shall be vulnerable in the way that is expected of us.

I think it is out of respect for this that some doctors are uneasy about telling patients the raw truth about their condition. They feel that by doing this they are laying a heavy load on to the shoulders of someone already weakened by disease. Certainly, in the case of a patient who is choosing to deny the seriousness of the situation, then negative information from the doctor would certainly be counter-productive.

In contrast to doctors who hold back information, there are others who do quite the reverse. I think one of the reasons that doctors are sometimes callously blunt in the way they tell patients that they can only expect to live a few months, is due to a deep anxiety about reprisals. When I once asked a hospital doctor why he didn't tell me all about the glittering success stories instead of pointing out the five year 'average' survival, he said, 'But you might not be one of those successes and then I would have misled you.' I asked him what he thought I would do if that proved to be the case. If I was dead and buried I could not easily come back full of revenge and recrimination. *He* was quite safe from negative outcomes, but the same was not true for me. When patients are given limited and prescribed horizons they tend to limit their hopes and expectations accordingly. They then run the risk of becoming a self-fulfilling prophesy rather than a self-actualizing person.

The present confusion over the patient's right to information has led to a glorious muddle. Half the patients who come to Bristol complain that they could never get a straight answer from anybody in hospital and resorted to bribing the nurses into telling them what was going on. The other half tell horror stories of trotting into out-patients expecting to pick up some iron tablets for anaemia, only to be told they have leukaemia and are not expected to see Christmas.

Naturally the outraged panic expressed by the second group is all the justification required for doctors who do not want to tell the truth to their patients. They say something along the lines that even people who think they want the truth cannot handle it in the event. The weakness in this argument is that patients get more than information when the doctor tells them about their cancer, they get this model of disease in general, and his fear and anxiety about cancer in particular, thrown in as well. Hermann Feifel in a paper entitled 'Physicians Consider Death' (Proceedings of the American Psychological Association Convention 1967) suggests that doctors are significantly more afraid of death than either healthy or sick people. Ivan Illich in *The Limits to Medicine* goes so far as to say that this could lead to the thesis that physicians are carriers of 'infectious fright'!

This is piercingly relevant to the patient's frame of mind because, in addition to this, the doctor has been trained in a model of disease that says that (a) cancer can only be dealt with by mechanistic or chemical assault from the outside, and (b) these techniques have an alarmingly high failure rate. In these circumstances it is difficult, if not impossible, for the doctor to impart anything but a sense of helplessness and victimization to the patient.

The situation is totally different with a doctor who operates from a broader base. Doctors who believe that cancer can and should be tackled from many different angles, some of which are entirely within the patients' capacity to control, are capable of imparting information without despair.

So it is in fact possible to resolve the apparent paradox of the patient wanting to know the truth, but not wanting to take on board at the same time a whole bundle of beliefs and expectations that the doctor holds which the patient may not hold and would be better off without anyway. Only in the holistic model is it possible to integrate the patient's need for information with the need to feel positive and hopeful about the future.

All this is most relevant to the role of positive visualization because part of the value of this activity is that it helps us to de-bug ourselves of the negative programming that we have been given.

One of our doctors at the Centre says that our first role as therapists is to return our patients to the state they were in when they only had the symptoms of their disease without the diagnosis. In other words, our first task is to help the patient recover from the diagnosis and the prognosis. Patients usually have far more trouble with these than with their physical symptoms.

Of course it is not only the doctor who spreads the doom and gloom. All cancer patients know how vulnerable they are to the negative expectations of family, friends, community and the world at large. Even if by dint of great personal endeavour you get on top of the situation and embark on a day of optimism and hope, you are unlikely to get far before someone greets you with 'Are you *sure* you're really feeling alright?' or 'I think it's so brave of you to put up such a good show', or 'Don't you think you ought to be taking it easy under the circumstances?' These remarks are examples of the subtle way society reinforces its corporate beliefs about cancer. They have the effect of reminding you what you should believe and pulling you into line with what everyone else believes. Less subtle, but no doubt just as effective, was a remark made to a patient who bounced back for a return visit to her consultant, full of hope and vitality, only to hear, 'Well, the thing is, you're not as healthy as you think you are'!

Against this very depressing and negative background the patient needs to create a new, alternate reality. He needs to give mind and body a different scenario to work with, one in which he is healing and recovering. The two best ways of doing this are by positive affirmations and visualization.

Positive affirmations

Perhaps the most famous proponent of these was the French doctor Emile Coué. I always raise a smile of recognition from one or two faces if I talk to a group about 'Day by day in every way I am getting better and better' or 'Little by little, day by day, I am getting better and better'.

Affirmations should be simple and easy to remember. I made my first pathetic attempts with the aid of Catherine Ponder's book *Healing Secrets of the Ages*. I say 'pathetic' because I was so low mentally and emotionally that my voice used to dry up and I used to burst into tears every time I tried to affirm anything strong and helpful. Fortunately I recognized this as a sure sign that I needed to continue and struggled on until I could say something nice to myself without collapsing in the attempt. I only realized much later that I was making things harder for myself because the affirmations were too long. Even if I could get half way through without crying I found I couldn't remember the next bit and had to keep referring to the book. My advice is to keep affirmations short and simple:

I am a whole and happy person.
I am a powerful person capable of healing myself.
There is nothing to be afraid of.
I am loved and cared for.
All will be well and all manner of things will be well.
The kingdom of heaven is within me.
Whatever the outcome of my hospital check-up my future will be more wonderful than my past.

Work out what it is that you most want to hear and then say that to yourself.

Whenever possible affirmations should be made out loud. This does not mean to say that you have to scare everyone out of the hospital waiting room or have people moving to another seat on the bus. At those times make the affirmations silently, but set aside specific times during the day when you can affirm in a strong, bold voice whatever you have chosen to inspire yourself with. You can do this at odd times of day – in the bath or at the traffic lights in the car.

(Elizabeth Khubler-Ross recommends using the car when you need a bit of privacy to do some of her exercises and I have already suggested discharging negative emotions there. Also, my autogenic teacher gave us lots of exercises to do in the car, as did the man who taught me meditation. I am rapidly coming to the conclusion that the vast majority of excursions into personal growth and development take place in motor cars and when we think we are watching someone humming along to Radio 1 she is more than likely doing her daily dozen as recommended by her therapist.)

Affirmations are the quickest and easiest way towards building a new, positive image for the body to work with. I admit that it may be difficult to say these things with conviction and determination when your head is full of fear and panic, but since an affirmation only takes a moment or two it is a good place to start. You may find it easier if you put some of these to music and sing them. One cancer patient keeps up a regular correspondence with me, offering her latest compositions. Here are two of her suggestions:

> My cancer cells are dissolving,
> My cancer cells are dissolving,
> My cancer cells are dissolving,
> And they'll never get a hold again.

To the tune of 'I'm Gonna Leave Old Durham Town:
(Visualization: cells dissolving like Alka Seltzers in a beautiful blue healing liquid.)

If you have a more classical bent, this is her suggestion for Beethoven's 9th – the choral song of joy:

> 'Day by day I
> Fight my cancer,
> I'll kill every rotten cell.
> One by one my
> Needle bursts them,
> I will soon be
> Fit and well.'

(Do cell-bursting with big darning needle visualization to this one.)

This is, word for word, what she has written to me. A good example of how patients take these ideas and make them work in very personal ways. This woman is making a marvellous recovery.

Visualization

The idea behind visualization is that we should conjure up a picture in our minds of the body healing itself and looking after itself.

In order to do this effectively we should first relax deeply and then allow our images to form and float around in our consciousness while we are detached from our everyday existence. Obviously this requires a little more time and patience than the affirmations. Our therapists at Bristol recommend that patients aim to do this for thirty minutes at a time, twice or three times a day. Much depends on the individual, of course. Some patients may be setting aside time for meditation as well and therefore only practise visualization once a day, or more frequently but for a shorter period.

We often find that people who find meditation difficult make a better start with excursions into altered states of consciousness through visualization. If the mind is very busy with thoughts, then visualization is a way of acknowledging that activity and using it constructively. When we meditate we are trying to still the mind, to ignore its thoughts, but when we visualize we are deliberately taking those thoughts and shaping them in a positive way.

The Simontons in their book, *Getting Well Again*, (see Suggested reading page 146) have made famous the idea of visualizing the white cells of the body as sharks and the tumour as a cauliflower. Obviously sharks can shred and devour cauliflowers without any difficulty, and the message that the body receives is that the white cells are attacking and destroying the cancer in just the same way. An image of this sort is both specific and aggressive. This may be ideal for patients with an active cancer in the form of a tumour, but is obviously less appropriate for patients with leukaemia, or patients who are working on staying well rather than getting well.

I think visualizations that mount a very specific attack on disease in this way are more suitable for patients tackling existing tumours or conditions. This is true if their cancer is untreatable or if they are currently receiving treatment for it. Such an image would be an excellent adjunct to radiotherapy or chemotherapy treatment and is often used in these circumstances. However, when treatment is complete and the original tumour or condition has been destroyed, it may not be wise to continue with a visualization that keeps the original image alive. It would be more appropriate, then, to visualize in a less specific and aggressive way. Picturing the white blood cells shimmering with light and bubbling through the body, sweeping away any unwanted malingering cancer cells, is the sort of image that people feel most comfortable with when they have no specific cancer sites but want to keep their defences on the alert.

In this, as with everything else, it is best to find your own personal technique. The problem with books about the subject is that people tend to try what was written in the book and then give up if they don't get along with it. I have never been able to visualize a white cell as a shark or a tumour as a cauliflower. Never. But that doesn't mean to say I can't visualize. If I want to address myself specifically to getting rid of cancer, then I make a mental picture of all my cancer cells piled up in front of me on a plate in the form of ice-cubes. I then take these and put them in the full glare of the sun in a beautiful garden and sit and watch them melt away. In the end it really doesn't matter what pictures or images you choose as long as you follow a few basic guidelines.

If you are using material images, like sharks and ice cubes, you must make sure that the cancer is represented by something that is weaker and less powerful than whatever image you have for your immune system. It is no good picturing your cancer as a rock that is being washed away by healing water. Healing water is a lovely image but it is no match for granite. This kind of attrition takes aeons of time. If you find yourself making the cancer stronger and more enduring than your immune system this is likely to be a reflection of your doubts about your ability to recover. Don't worry about this, just give yourself a different picture. The encounter that you are going to conjure up every day must be between a mighty, powerful force and a weak, feeble opposition. If you like the feeling that you get from an image of healing water, then by all means use it, but adjust your image of the tumour to sandcastles that are washed smooth by the incoming tide.

Don't leave the job half finished. Each time you embark on a session of visualization always end it with the cancer completely overcome and swept away. Some patients find this hard to do because they are glaringly aware of the fact that the cancer has not gone away. It is still palpable and painful, and they are acutely conscious of it. Nevertheless we encourage patients to do this. To finish up with a mental picture of being clear and free of disease. We believe that this is important on levels other than the physical. We shall all be completely healed in a spiritual sense, whether or not we get rid of disease. But it may also be important to the body for us to conceptualize the possibility of perfection. If we never offer it this potential we are imposing our own limitations on what it can do. In a funny kind of way we are saying 'You can get a little bit better, but you can't get completely better'. This is just another version of the negative expectations we are receiving from other people. No, we must go all the way with this, and allow our visualizations to be completely successful.

Although I shall give a few examples of possible visualization techniques, it is much better to arrive at one's own. Be completely open-minded about this, don't resist anything, however odd and unlikely it may sound. Our experience at Bristol is that patients find it much easier to work with their own images than one suggested by somebody else. Perhaps one of the most unusual was the lady with the Golden Hoover. Her visualization consisted of directing this magic machine to buzz all around her body sucking up all the dirt and rubbish and unwanted debris from every possible nook and cranny. Fascinated by this, one of our doctors asked her, 'How do you start? I mean, where do you keep it?'

'Oh, I don't keep it anywhere. I leave it running all the time, so I actually have to go and find it before I begin.'

By this simple device she had programmed into her scheme the idea that the healing/Hoovering was going on *all the time* and not just when she was visualizing it.

If this sounds all too complicated and fussy for words then it would be a good idea to start with the simplest visualization of them all: imagining yourself well. This can be done in the form of an elaborate day-dream. Perhaps you will find yourself picking up glimpses of the way you used to do this as a child. Nearly all of us can recall day-dreaming about our future as an engine-driver, a world-famous ballerina, scoring the deciding goal in the World Cup, or just breaking away from home into a place of our own.

Some people, to begin with, find it hard to visualize

themselves well in the future, so they start by remembering themselves well in the past. If you do this often enough you will soon find that you can start projecting into the future, conjuring up a vital and appealing picture of yourself. I encourage patients to incorporate specific goals into this future projection.

Goals

Setting goals is a form of positive visualization. If you are determined to live long enough to give your daughter away at her wedding then you are capable of visualizing yourself doing this. Work on this image. You are not going to totter up the aisle and ruin everyone's day with your pallor, you are going to have a new suit and amaze them all by looking wonderful in the photographs.

Most of us will have adjusted our ambitions from the day-dreaming, bee-loud days of hot sunny classrooms. We have probably given up the idea of taking seventeen curtain calls at Covent Garden, but are we still harbouring a longing to have singing lessons? I found that the shock of the diagnosis catapulted me into thinking about all the things I had hoped and planned to do, but had never got around to. While I was still a novice in the healing arts of meditation and visualization I was quite capable of setting myself the goal of fulfilling small ambitions. I encouraged myself to imagine a future where I was skimming across a lake on a wind-surfer, and by doing this I was learning to use a goal as a method of positive visualization.

One of my favourite of these visualizations is to imagine myself as a very old lady. Someone pottering around the garden, not eating regular meals, only bothering to answer the phone when I feel like, watching the antics of my children with detached tolerance.

The advantage of simply visualizing yourself well and healthy and happy in the future is that this may expose feelings that you have about yourself that you are not conscious of.

When we first started the Centre one of our earliest patients was a girl with lung secondaries following a breast cancer. She was enthusiastic about what Bristol had to offer, was a vigorous and faithful devotee of the diet, had her doctor running around prescribing all the vitamins and minerals, and was generally a model patient. Unfortunately she did not seem to be much better for all this, and we were concerned about her lack of progress.

She came to us one week wanting some specific advice about her visualizations. These took the form of a very clinical, pathological battle between T-lymphocytes and cancer cells and she came bearing medical text books full of blown-up, magnified colour pictures of all these cells. She had a very technical discussion with the doctor, but as she was leaving something made me say to her:

'Something else you might try is a short visualization where you just imagine yourself well.'

I don't think any of us was prepared for what happened next. She *burst* into tears. She gave meaning to the phrase. One minute she was smiling goodbye to the doctor and myself, the next her face had crumpled and tears were splashing from her eyes. She almost shouted at me:

'Oh no! I could never do that.'

During the discussion that followed it became clear that this girl had such a low self-image that she couldn't allow herself to do such a thing as picture herself well and happy. I believe that if people have such a low self-image that they cannot even *imagine* themselves better, then no amount of treatment in the world can help them. Fortunately this revelation enabled the girl to work more directly and openly with her counsellor who helped her to feel better about herself and her right to live, and she began to improve almost at once.

Some ideas for visualization
Settle yourself for your visualization session following the instructions on relaxation on page 108–110.

Add intention.

Your intention this time is to picture your body healing itself. Remind yourself that you are capable of seeking out unwanted cells, breaking them up and getting rid of them. Now imagine that your white cells, the ones that are designed to do this, are beautiful, clean white goats. They are gentle and benign creatures, but they are quick on their feet, agile and fast-moving. They are moving throughout your body eating up all the rubbish. They have a preference for unwanted growth, just in the way a goat will eat the nettles in preference to the grass in an orchard. They have strong horns which they can use to break up and tear into any big tangles of weeds and junk. Their mouths are so tough they can chew, and apparently enjoy, even sharp brambles. There is nothing unwanted they cannot devour and recycle to a harmless pulp. Once the goats have eaten your cancer cells they are rendered harmless and destroyed.

You can either picture the goats at work in your body, or imagine that your body is a meadow or an orchard and put them to work there. Remember these goats are brilliant white and have no enemies. When the tumour has gone or the meadow is neat and tidy with only lovely flowers and trees growing there, leave the goats grazing and come back to full awareness.

A completely different kind of visualization would be to move your attention from your breathing to the beating of your heart and imagine your blood surging around your body. Picture your blood containing little sparkling flashes of white light which are increasing in number all the time. These are your white cells preparing themselves for action. Soon your blood is so full of these glittering, shiny sparkles of white that it is no longer red, but pulsing with bright light. This light is reaching into every part of you, even those backwaters where dark cancer cells are stagnating. The dull, murky cancer cells are surrounded by the white sparkling blood, they are buffeted and washed by this swilling, healing stream, and they are transformed. The healing, white, dancing power in your blood is indestructible. Nothing can stand in its way. Everything is being washed and cleansed and becoming beautiful and wholesome again.

Continue doing this until all images of darkness, all lumpy black masses, all messy impure corners have been swept away. Watch the jumping, bubbling stream of white sparkles gradually quieten down and reduce in number until your blood appears as red again. Red healthy blood carrying a few of the white, sun-bright dancers who are permanently on duty, always watching and checking and keeping you pure and safe.

Since the idea of visualization is to use an image or a picture to carry a message I often suggest people do this when they are *not* relaxing. You can use a similar technique when you are going about your usual day-to-day tasks. If you are gardening, focus your mind for a moment or two on the idea of the weed you are pulling up being a cancer cell. As you clear and aerate the soil, imagine your body doing the same thing. Just do this for a moment or two, then return to the job in the usual way. You could equally well imagine your body being cleansed of cancer each time you hold a dirty plate under a running tap, or clean the bath, or put a load of washing in the machine. If you go for a walk in the country, let nature do the work. Watch the sheep tirelessly cropping the grass and think of your scavenger cells eating away at your cancer. These momentary flash-pictures will all help to build up a healing scenario for your body to work with.

Suggested reading
Getting Well Again by Carl and Stephanie Simonton (Bantam Books).

4

Beyond Belief

CREATIVITY

The verb 'to create' has several senses: 'to bring into existence'; 'to originate'; 'to give rise to'; 'to produce by what one does'; 'to give a new rank or position'; 'to make a fuss or grumble'. Not all these meanings are associated with the adjective 'creative' which the Oxford dictionary describes as: 'Having the power or ability to create things ... showing imagination and originality ...'

This is the meaning that we are interested in. It is rather unfortunate that most people are attached to the idea that creativity means producing something. That at the end of creative activity there will be some kind of concrete, tangible thing, a sort of evidence or proof that something creative really happened.

Most understandably this inhibits many people, driving them into believing that, because they can't paint something worth framing or sew something fit to wear, then they are not capable of being creative. It is ironic really that the kind of creativity we are hoping to evoke in patients at Bristol is definitely not goal-orientated in this way, but the average person is locked into this way of thinking. As soon as we mention Art Therapy there are cries of 'but I'm hopeless at drawing!' Remarks like this and 'I'm no good at anything artistic', reflect the fact that most people judge the activity of doing something in terms of its end product. This is hardly surprising when seen in the context of the kind of schooling most of us have experienced. After a couple of terms having a wonderful time messing about in the art room and eating the drawing charcoal I was told I had to 'give up art' because I didn't show any natural talent. I was quite surprised by this. I thought I had bags of talent because I was enjoying it all so much, but it was soon pointed out to me that the feeling of contentment and pleasure that hummed through me on Wednesday afternoons was not the object of the exercise. I fared a little better in the choir and was only a witness, not a victim, to the scene of my tone-deaf pals being firmly ejected.

The kind of creativity I am talking about is to do with performance and experience, not production: the process, not the event. At Bristol we are interested in the last of the above definitions – 'showing imagination and originality' – which is a style of behaving, not a means to an end. In short we are talking about self-expression: the ability to experience who we are through creative, pleasurable activity.

It is hardly surprising that we should all have become obsessed with the idea of creativity being productive because our cultural background, and that of many other countries, is buzzing with the demands of the work ethic. In the case of the United Kingdom, America and most of Europe, we are stuck, not only with the idea that productive work is good and desirable, but, thanks to the grip of the Protestant ethic, that it is in some way 'morally right' as well. It is but a short step from here to the view that there is something wrong with non-productive activity.

Most people feel guilty doing nothing. Small wonder. Most of us have been drilled into feeling that way. I have to make a conscious effort not to call upstairs and demand of an unusually silent teenager 'I hope you're doing something useful up there?'

Why should everyone always be doing something, useful or otherwise? Why do I find it difficult to let my children 'hang out' or 'mess about'? Two reasons. One is that my mother wouldn't let me and this is a hard pattern to break, the other is that the kind of activity that produces something – like a string of 'O' levels or grade 6 clarinet – gives me the proof I need that I am a good mother. Most of us are tangled up in this, both with regard to our expectations of others and ourselves. Doing is fine: being makes us nervous. Creativity is about being, not doing.

Even if we are lucky enough to be allowed to dabble in areas of pleasurable contentment this doesn't usually last for long. If we learn to play the piano and sit pottering away at it, we shall soon hear the voice from the kitchen saying, 'It's such a pity you didn't work hard at that and take it up seriously, you could have been really good at it.'

This must cause terrible confusion in the mind of one who is thoroughly enjoying the experience of playing around with music, being creative in the sense of being imaginative and original and self-expressive, but because it is not goal-orientated it is briskly discouraged.

If we are going to start being creative and express ourselves in a non-productive sense we shall have to begin by allowing ourselves to do it. We have to countermand years of training that says this kind of activity is 'a waste of time' and give ourselves permission.

What exactly am I suggesting you should do?

I have to tread very carefully here because this is such a personal thing. Some cancer patients can identify very clearly with thwarted and frustrated creative ambitions. There are areas of their lives that cry out for attention, activities just longing to be pursued. All that is required is that they should be allowed to spend time doing the things they want to do. Finding an outlet for their creativity is not a problem, letting themselves indulge in it is the barrier.

These barriers are built up in part by our political and social environment but as individuals we also help to maintain them. When a person develops cancer something interesting happens – a lot of the social and domestic barriers come down. Because of the fear and awe with which society regards the disease of cancer, it affords considerable indulgence to the people who suffer from it. This was certainly my experience.

Almost overnight I found that the people around me were a lot more accommodating to my wishes. In this respect cancer had its positive side. I was soon to learn that there were other side-effects of the diagnosis that I quite enjoyed. This is covered more closely in the chapter 'How To Start Helping Yourself' but it comes under the heading of Secondary Gains. One of the spin-offs of having cancer is that the social pressures on you are likely to be lifted. If you announce that you are taking up pot-holing or pottery you are less likely to be greeted with remarks like, 'It's all very well for some' or 'I don't know where you find the time for these things'.

Such remarks, which are intended to pull you back into line with all the restraints operating against the speaker, are entirely inappropriate in relation to someone who may not be long for this world. Since this belief is part of the built-in stereotype that most people have of cancer patients you may find that your friends, family and neighbours are a lot more tolerant of your behaviour than you might have expected.

So, if they are not going to give you any trouble, what's the problem? You are, I expect. Your 'internal saboteur' is flexing his muscles. Week after week at Bristol I hear people say that they think it would be 'selfish' to do something that they enjoy, just for its own sake, regardless of whether it is useful or important. Selfish is right. But not the narrow, exclusive, thoughtless 'selfish' – more a reasonable attention to the needs and wants of the self. There is nothing wrong in this. More to the point, it is essential.

Creativity may be our way in to releasing a whole new and untapped healing potential within us. It may be a way of redirecting pent up energies that are festering away as a cancer.

The medical definition of cancer is 'neo-plasm'. This means 'new growth'. A feature of cancer cells is that they proliferate in a crazy and uncontrolled fashion. They keep reproducing themselves, they form clusters and start creating new, un-wanted structures. Supposing these neo-plasms, or new growths, are developing as a result of suppressed growth at another level? Carl Jung obviously thought along these lines, talking about cancer as unlived life.

I know that this will be an extraordinary idea for some people to grasp, but stay with it for a minute. We are being forced to accept that the old medical paradigm of curing cancer by getting rid of its physical manifestation via external forces is just not working. As soon as we expand the medical model, and admit that other factors and forces might be instrumental in our susceptibility to the disease and our recovery from it, then we must be prepared to look at all possibilities.

The traditional Chinese model of disease, with which I am most familiar, would have no difficulty in accepting this idea. If energy is suppressed and stifled it will not just go away. It will either become polluted or the excessive build-up will give rise to symptoms. The idea of physical symptoms arising from causative factors beyond the body is axiomatic to the Chinese model.

We have seen that it is not hard to understand ways in which a person's creative life force can be suppressed. The work of suppressing it continues tirelessly in competitive educational establishments, in ambitious homes and families, and in high-production factories. Many cancer patients have been barred from, or forbidden access to, ways of being that they once delighted in. Wordsworth wrote:

> Though nothing can bring back the hour
> Of splendour in the grass, of glory in the flower;

but I think he is wrong. That is exactly what we can and must do.

At Bristol we offer people a few opportunities of releasing their own creative side. We have two art therapists, one who is trained in the Rudolph Steiner anthroposophical school, and another who takes a different approach. Between them they spend time with all our residential patients and as many day patients as possible, but we are severely limited by the restrictions of a very short week. We would love to do more with movement and music, but, rather than try to present creative outlets for patients, we try to help them discover their own. We suggest to them the possibility that they might have a great deal of unexpressed energy that may be fermenting away as a cancer for want of any proper outlet.

Naturally this idea is greeted with enthusiasm by some but creates a degree of puzzled uncertainty in others. You may be one of the lucky ones who, on reflection, can think of lots of ways in which your style of being, your way of humming happily along in the world, has been discouraged or forbidden. In this case you have only to move into these areas and allow yourself to explore them. If your mother or some other authoritarian figure wouldn't let you, then give yourself permission. Start now. Buy a box of paints, a recorder, a bicycle and start enjoying yourself.

If you are one of the people who can't think of anything in particular that you want to do, and you don't know where to start, start with that last phrase – 'enjoying yourself'. Enjoying your *self*. You may find you can do this lying on the grass, squinting up at the sunlight through the trees. Remember, this kind of creativity does not require an end product. It requires only that you give yourself an outlet for being who you are. Sometimes it helps to recapture times in our childhood when we did this with relative ease. An absolutely sure-fire, guaranteed way for me to feel totally in harmony with myself and what I am doing is to have a go on a playground swing. I am then immediately transported to a time in my life when playing was the expression of myself. Play. Not work, or good deeds, or fancy clothes, or a seat on the board. How long since you did something you enjoyed for no other reason than that you enjoy doing it? That's the kind of painting I was doing in the art room, that's the kind of creativity I mean. It's called playing.

Lin Yutang says in his book *The Awakening*:

Probably the Creator knew well that, when he created man upon this earth, he was producing a scamp, a brilliant scamp it is true, but a scamp nonetheless. The scamp-like qualities of man are, after all, his most hopeful qualities.

Scamps are mischievous and playful, and playing, by definition, is fun. Things that are fun make you laugh, and laughter is good for you. Nobody demonstrates this better than Norman Cousins in his book *Anatomy of Illness*. He claims that a combination of vitamin C and a lot of laughing helped him to recover from a very serious disease. I am particularly fond of this book because it is the hardest thing in the world to laugh when you are struggling with a serious illness, and Cousins shows us that we may have to resort to tactics when spontaneity is beyond us. His tactic was to get hold of a projector and watch all his favourite funny films. In the world of video recorders this would be a relatively easy thing to do, but first we have to allow ourselves to do this.

As soon as we start trying to have a good time, doing creative, funny things, we come up against the boring but familiar mind-sets of society's expectations of cancer patients. They have it in mind that we should be addressed in hushed and lowered tones and spend half our life in bed being miserable. When I finally achieved my goal of standing up long enough on a wind-surfer to claim to be in control of it, one of my acquaintances said, 'But I thought you were meant to have cancer.'

I admit it isn't easy, but if we keep at it long enough, not only do we change the way we feel about ourselves, we change the way other people respond to us. I have been fascinated over the years at the power we have to alter, not just our own perception of reality, but that of the people around us. My second stay in hospital was markedly different from my first because in the intervening years I had worked hard at *not* being a typical cancer patient. This had led to a situation where the doctors who gathered around the end of my bed were almost as interested in my monkey-brown hands, tanned to perfection on a recent cycling holiday, as they were in my rather peculiar-looking left breast. As a result of this everyone was a great deal more cheerful and positive than I expected. My consultant said he thought this was all a false alarm, and he was sure there was nothing malignant in these lumps and bumps. Even when his investigations proved this not to be the case, he was free with encouraging remarks about how I seemed to be on top of it. I found that my determined efforts to lead a happy and fulfilling, and at times rather silly, life – one that cut across their expectations of a cancer patient – had brought me to the point where my medical team had stopped treating me like one.

I have heard the same from many Bristol patients. As the weeks, months and years go by they alter the behaviour and expectations of everyone around them by their own example. How lovely that we can do this just as effectively through enjoyment, creativity and laughter as by effort and will.

'The scamp will be the champion of human dignity and individual freedom, and will be the last to be conquered.'

Ideas about letting go of repressions and denials and allowing ourselves to express freely may seem rather remote from the cancer crisis, but there are other systems of medicine where this is not so. Older civilizations than ours believe that disease is the result of our intellect, mind and ego becoming so over-developed and dense, that the spirit of the higher self cannot filter through. They believe that when this imbalance occurs disease will be the automatic consequence. This is only another way of warning us not to stop being creative. Our working definition of creative is 'showing imagination and originality' and what is originality if not that part of ourselves that is unique – our higher or true self? If we can open up the channels that connect us to this part of ourselves we may be taking an important step towards healing.

Professor Nixon and Dr Hywell Williams are using dancing as a creative activity in the treatment of heart patients. This important and exciting work is going on at the centre of Charing Cross Hospital. They use music and masks to help patients develop and experience their creativity.

One of the things I learned during the course of using bio-feedback is that we have two hemispheres in our brains that are quite separate, although they work together. If you watch your brainwaves flickering away on a screen in front of you, you may notice that one side is busier than the other. It is widely believed that the left side of the brain (that controls the right side of the body) is the part that we use when we calculate, work things out logically, and plot and plan generally. Conversely, the right side of the brain (which controls the left side of the body) is the part we use when we experience the world through our senses and feelings in an intuitive, spontaneous way. Most of us tend to favour left brain activity, and have developed this side of ourselves at the expense of our more creative, intuitive feeling side. Only when the two are in balance and harmony can we be said to be well and healthy.

The trouble is that we are in something of a Catch 22 situation here. The harder we try to gain access to the right side of our brain the less likely we are to succeed because 'trying' is a left-brain activity. Neither is it possible to open up the right side of our brain by learning any special techniques because the learning process itself is a left brain activity! To do this we must use our feelings and our senses, not our intellect and our thoughts. Rudolph Steiner encouraged his cancer patients to experiment with paint (colour) and clay (sensation). One of the best ways to wake up our right-brain potential is to be creative and spontaneous. It is only when we stop thinking about it and start experiencing it that an activity reaches us in this way. T. S. Eliot speaks of

> music heard so deeply
> That it is not heard at all, but you are the music
> While the music lasts.
>
> 'Four Quartets'

Art therapy is one of the ways we help patients to deal with their intuition rather than their reason.

Once we have managed to convince everyone that art therapy is not our way of collecting pictures to hang in the lounge, and that artistic ability in this respect might even be a disadvantage, everyone has a thoroughly good time messing about with paints. Sometimes the therapist will suggest a theme and often this will have direct relevance to what is going on in the patient's life. The picture can be painted in blobs and squiggles and symbols and interpreted later. 'This mushy bit over here is how I think my family see me; this tiny little stick insect is how I feel about myself.' After some slight, initial embarrassment, patients generally have a wonderful time in the art room and thoroughly enjoy themselves. Oddly enough this is still true even when painting releases suppressed negative emotions, as it often does. Only a few weeks ago a patient left the art room weeping. She said she had not cried for five years. During that time her husband had left her and her son had died of cancer and she herself had been diagnosed, but she had not cried once. She was grateful to the art therapist and went back for more.

Sometimes the act of operating through our senses, by seeing shapes rather than words, colours instead of objects, we open ourselves up to parts of our existence that have been locked away. An Australian woman came to Bristol last year. She had a strong personality and a fairly assertive style. One day I listened while she told me and a group of patients what she thought of art therapy.

First of all she didn't want to go at all. She thought art therapy was a silly waste of time. She hadn't come all the way from Australia to mess about with paper and paints, and she was annoyed that anyone should suggest such a thing. But then she decided she was paying good money for this, so she would make herself go, but she wouldn't join in. She was already cross and frustrated when she arrived at the art room and immediately became even more furious because the therapist had not arrived. Fuming with rage she told us how she snatched up a brush and scrabbled out some kind of painting which she promptly screwed up into a ball and threw into the waste-paper basket. At this point the therapist arrived. He retrieved her scrumpled-up paper from the basket and smoothed it out on the table with the words 'let's look at what part of yourself you're so quick to throw away'.

Within minutes this angry woman had melted into a little girl again. She told us how she had drawn an image of her mother, and that what she had thrown away was a childhood of disappointments and lack of love. She started to recall things she had not given a thought to for over thirty years. She knew she had unfinished business with her mother and that this had distorted her relationship with her own children. She ended by telling us that after this experience she knew exactly what she wanted to talk to her counsellor about, that the rest of her stay in Bristol had become very exciting and happy. She said she was no longer afraid of having cancer, it might even have been necessary for her to have it. She couldn't wait to get back to Australia and take up her old life with her new self.

She said she would not have achieved any of this if she had not gone to the art room.

It was one of the most exciting and moving testimonials I have ever heard. All the more so because she shared, with such humour, her initial resistance to the thought of art therapy. This is a phenomenon I have witnessed more than once. Where there is strong resistance to any aspect of therapy it is almost as if the will is deliberately blocking what it knows will be a successful route to wholeness. Perhaps because the will and intellect have ruled the roost for so long there is a special reluctance to let go. Whatever the reason, when patients say they had to overcome a good deal of prejudice about something, they are more than likely to admit that the very same thing led to a breakthrough for them, and has become an important part of their lives.

Once we allow ourselves to side-step the barriers of

prejudice and admit that creativity may be part of the healing process, and that lack of it may have contributed to our disease, then we can avail ourselves of a wide range of healing potential. It is not always necessary to work with professionals in order to do this. Certainly there are people who are experts in the use of colour or sound as therapy, but joining a painting class or singing in the church choir can be just as potent. Although professionals may help in the beginning, they would be the first to say that it is only when self-expression and creativity become part of our everyday existence, that it can be truly said to be healing.

If your family complain about your singing in the bath every night, tell them you're reactivating your right brain. They'll understand.

Suggested reading
The Psychology of Consciousness by Robert Ornstein (Pelican).
Art Therapy for Groups by Marian Liebmann (Croom Helm).

HEALING

When the Cancer Help Centre first started we were offered the use of a house where healing was already taking place. Canon Christopher Pilkington and his wife Pat were actively involved in a ministry of healing long before they became involved with the Centre. This meant that our first home was a place of prayer already, and we benefited greatly as a result of this. There was a room in the building where healing had been offered with prayer and the laying on of hands, and the feeling of power and spirit that surrounded this room helped us in our work there. When it became obvious a few years later that we would have to find new premises I don't think any of us could believe that we would be this lucky again; but we were.

Grove House was once a convent, and the room there which

we use for healing was once the nuns' chapel. The atmosphere in this room is almost palpable. There is a feeling of strength and peace that is both restful and inspiring; there is an air of spirituality that is both soothing and empowering. This beautiful atmosphere has built up during the many years that the room has been used for the purposes of prayer and praise, and the sanctification and administration of the communion host. One after the other the directors looking around the building fell under the almost hypnotic spell of this room. We admitted this to each other later and at different times, but we were immediately unanimous in our decision to buy Grove House.

The nuns too were pleased that their chapel should be put to what they considered to be such good use, and they departed with the promise to continue praying for us. Years later I met one of them on a retreat. She recognized me, and before she left she told me that she had never failed to remember us, and every one of our patients, daily. It is wonderful to know that there is a mighty prayer wheel turning out there on our behalf.

It is quite obvious from this that the Centre has its roots in the Christian tradition. We were aware from the beginning that this rather formal, 'churchy' association might create difficulties for some people. In fact we were so sensitive to this possibility that we even discussed the idea of playing it down; not letting our Christian petticoats show, you might say. Looked at in that way it soon seemed pretty ridiculous. After all we are talking about spirituality, not denominationalism. If I was visiting a centre in Israel I would expect it to have its roots in Judaism; in India I would expect Hinduism, and so on. This would not amaze or alarm me; quite the contrary, I should be delighted. It would show me that someone was flying the flag for man as a spiritual being in the way he knew best. For the co-founders at Bristol, Christianity is our way, our chosen path, but we would never want this to be a stumbling block for others. At the beginning of his book *Wellsprings*, the Jesuit writer de Mello says: 'In spite of frequent references to Jesus Christ, whose disciple the author professes himself to be, this book is meant for persons of all affiliations – religious, a-religious, agnostic, atheistic.' (See Suggested reading, page 166). These are my feelings exactly in writing about spiritual healing. My background and bias are Christian but this is not so for many of our staff.

We have such a wide variety of spiritual beliefs represented by the staff at Bristol I think it would be impossible for anyone to feel out of place or uncomfortable there. Morning prayers are said in the chapel every day, but this is not a stiffly structured service, and it has been happily attended over the years by Moslems, Jews, Buddhists, agnostics, and – would you believe it – atheists. Obviously we are not an exclusively Christian organization.

All this is most relevant to a discussion about healing. Not just because the chapel becomes the healing room by the flick of a card, but because of the people who work there. Not all of our healers are priests, and not all of them are Christians. We thought that some people might find the idea of spiritual healing difficult to swallow, especially if they were not themselves religious, so it seemed wise to have some healers with no particular affiliation. We were right about that. Equally, some people might have felt they could not receive healing from someone who was not ordained, so we also have healers who are priests. We were right about that too. We also thought there would be people who did not want healing at all, in any shape or form. We were wrong about that.

I have been asking around the Centre to see if anyone there can remember a patient who refused to have healing. There appear to be one or two people that the staff are not sure about, which, out of a total of nearly four thousand patients is amazing. Our experience is that patients are almost unanimous, both in their wish to have healing, and in their enthusiasm for its effects.

Inevitably something entitled 'spiritual healing' invites the supposition that the healing that takes place will be healing of the spirit. I am quite sure that healing of this kind does indeed occur, but we cannot rule out the idea that healing can take place at other levels too. In this respect healing has the same characteristic as other aspects of the Bristol Programme; on the surface it appears to be aimed at one particular part of the whole person, but it frequently influences other aspects as well.

I have known many patients who have experienced comfort from pain; patients who have gained a great increase in physical energy; and even a few who have believed that healing has helped their cancer to diminish.

There are others who take from the healing session a greater clarity of mind; they feel stronger mentally and emotionally; they feel empowered. For others the experience is entirely spiritual. They feel loved and forgiven and unafraid. They feel closer to God and more aware of themselves as a spiritual being. I have yet to meet the person who didn't feel they benefited at all.

Hopefully this will have dealt with the popular misconception that you have to be religious to have healing. You don't. Now let's look at some other questions and areas of confusion.

Do you have to believe in it?

A reasonable question since some people prefer to talk about 'faith healing' in this context. No you don't. Years ago a healer friend of mine, famous for jamming the switchboard at Pebble Mill with enquiries after a brief TV appearance, told me. '*You* don't have to have faith, but I have to have faith. I believe for you.' They were delivering his mail in sacks for months. There is a great hunger for the spiritual in this material world.

So don't be put off by your own lack of faith. Without getting trapped in a lot of theological debate it is worth saying that 'faith' and 'belief' are not quite the same thing. Saint Mark tells us the story of a leper who approached Jesus for help : 'If you want to,' he said, 'you can cure me.' Feeling sorry for him Jesus stretched out his hand and touched him. 'Of course I want to!' he said. 'Be cured!' And the leprosy left him at once and he was cured. (Mark 1: 40–42)

This man did not show the slightest doubt that Jesus could heal him. He believed and he had faith. However, many of us are riddled with doubts and fears that make us hold back from the act of crying out for help. In these circumstances belief is beyond us, but we can still hope. In his letter to the Hebrews, Paul describes faith in terms of hope. Hope may be all we can offer at the beginning, but it is enough. If our hope leads us to seek help we are on the way towards faith. In the meantime we can lean into the faith of others.

Do healers touch you?

Not necessarily. Again, since healing is often referred to as 'the laying on of hands' you might expect this, but generally that phrase relates to the priestly act of blessing and anointing with oil. Some healers do touch you, but there is no need for them to, and if you prefer not to be touched you should say so. I used to find it appropriate for my healer to put his hands where I was feeling pain, but others might find this disturbing. Healers all have their own style, but they would not need to touch you in order to help you. Indeed some of them prefer to work with their hands held a few inches from the body.

Sometime healers are working on your aura. This is an energy field that some very sensitive people can actually see in glowing colours surrounding the body. Other healers may be concentrating on chakras which are specific, but separate, energy fields that we all have but are often unaware of. Restoring harmony and balance in these energy fields will often lead to a wholeness and harmony in the physical body.

Do healers give you something specific, or pass something into you?

Sometimes patients feel warmth and tingling when they

receive healing, almost like a mild electric current, but the healer is not doing this – you are. Because healers all work in their own way and may come from diverse spiritual traditions they also talk about their work in different ways. But one thing they all agree about is that they themselves do very little. They see themselves as being channels through which healing energy can flow. This means they help you to be more receptive to healing forces that are gifts of the spirit and freely available to us all.

Some healers have no interest in auras or chakras but concentrate entirely on interceding between the patient and God. Both techniques lead to the same end. Healers know that they themselves do nothing; all healing comes from God.

Will they ask a lot of questions?

Almost certainly not. Unlike other activities at Bristol which require the patient to work very hard, healing is a passive therapy and comes as a blissful oasis of peace in an otherwise busy week. Naturally any healer is going to show an intelligent and friendly interest in what is happening to you, but you don't have to engage in a wordy encounter, or have what amounts to a consultation before treatment.

Does it cost a lot of money?

Most healers do not charge at all for their services. This is remarkable really since many of them provide comfortable premises in their own home, and devote a great deal of time to their work. Sometimes they will accept a donation or a contribution towards their expenses.

What am I likely to feel?

Having just said healing is a fairly passive activity I am now going to say that you could feel a bit emotional. Some people might find that they cry a little, but that this is not in the least bit distressing. Indeed this would be a powerful releasing of tension, a clearing away of something that might have been a barrier to healing. I once astonished myself and my healer by bursting out laughing; an unforgettable moment – I feel good just thinking about it. You may have sensations of warmth or heat or tingling. You may just feel pleasantly relaxed. Some people are so relaxed by healing that they feel tired afterwards and maybe even fall asleep. You may not feel anything at all at the time, but that does not mean that nothing is happening.

The Christian tradition has always had close links with healing and many churches hold healing services on a regular basis. You don't have to be a member of the church in order to go to a service and it is something that you might try. Some of these services are very powerful indeed, and we can learn a lot about healing by studying the ministry and service of Jesus.

We know from the healing stories in the New Testament that Jesus's healings were not all the same. He knew that different people needed different things. On one occasion He mixed up a clay and applied it like a poultice to the sufferer. With this symbolic gesture I think He is acknowledging the fact that some of us need to see outward signs that show we are being looked after, and also He is showing us how the physical and the spiritual can work together in the healing process.

> After spitting on the man's eyes, Jesus placed his hands on him and asked him, 'Can you see anything?'
>
> The man looked up and said, 'Yes, I can see people, but they look like trees walking about.'
>
> Jesus again placed his hands on the man's eyes. This time the man looked intently, his eyesight returned, and he saw everything clearly. (Mark 8: 23–25)

We can learn something else that is very important from this story; that healing may not be instantaneous. It is quite obvious from Bible readings that most of Jesus's healings were effected instantly and because of this I am fascinated by the message of this particular incident. Here we are told in a most graphic and poetic way that the blind man needed more than one healing or treatment. The first time Jesus ministered to him he improved, but the job was still only half done; he needed Jesus to lay his hands on him again.

Jesus was the word become flesh, dwelling among us; the son of the living God, and yet in this story he is showing us that healing may be a process and not an event. How much more true is this likely to be of *our* efforts? We should not despair if the healing seems slow. We may need to return time and again to the source before we feel ourselves responding to its power. Our healers at Bristol encourage patients to contact the National Federation of Spiritual healers and go for healing on a regular basis, twice or even three times a week.

In contrast to this story we have others that show a direct link between suffering and guilt. Jesus often assured the sick that their sins were forgiven and this was all that was needed for physical healing to take place. Here again we are being reminded that one cannot sensibly isolate man's feelings and emotions from his physical body. We have on occasions had patients at Bristol who felt they were unworthy of receiving healing, and this is a reflection of the same deep sense of shame that Jesus was so frequently aware of. Guilt is certainly a barrier to healing, one that needs to be dealt with as quickly as possible. Lacking Jesus's authority we deal with guilt through counselling, psychology, psychiatry, and through our own capacity to give unconditional love. But there will always be people who need forgiveness through the channel of confession.

Do whatever feels right for you. If you are a member of a church you could speak to your minister. There are many healing services and rituals that even regular worshippers know nothing about. Ask your community to pray for you. Pray for yourself. Find out about healing services in your neighbourhood. Above all try to incorporate spiritual healing into your life as a regular part of your existence. When you use diet as a healing adjunct you make it part of your everyday experience of the world; you don't starve all week and have an orgy of eating on Sunday. The same should be true of spiritual healing; open yourself to the possibility of spiritual healing being available to you all the time and it will soon become a reality.

For information about healers in your area contact:

The National Federation of Spiritual Healers
Old Manor Farm Studio
Church Street
Sunbury-on-Thames
Middx TW16 6RG

If you are Jewish contact:

L. E. Fowles
14 Gresham Road
Bournemouth

Suggested reading
Wellsprings by Anthony de Mello (Diaz del Rio S. J.)
The Power to Heal and *Healing*, by Francis MacNutt (Ave Maria Press).

5

Where Do We Go From Here?

'Search for *the* causes may be a hopeless pursuit because most disease states are the direct outcome of a constellation of circumstances rather than the direct result of single determinant factors.' *René Dubos, Mirage of Health*

HOW TO START HELPING YOURSELF

Obviously this chapter, like all the others, is written in a way that assumes the reader has cancer. However I hope it will be read by people who do not have cancer, and who would like to take whatever steps they can towards not only avoiding ever having cancer, but to achieving their maximum health potential. Everything about the Bristol Programme, and all the exercises suggested in this book, are entirely suitable as preventive measures. This would be a good re-evaluation programme for anyone.

Before you start on your healing journey buy an attractive notebook to work in. Make this simple act a gesture to yourself. Buy something a bit smarter and nicer than you might have done, something that will please you every time you look at it. Its initial purpose will be for jotting down notes about yourself as you do the following exercises, but it is always sensible to have a place to record the titles of good books that people recommend, the telephone numbers of interesting organizations, therapists and so on.

The problem with an holistic approach to healing is that it is sometimes a bit difficult to know where to start. If you are lucky you will have an inclination towards a particular source of healing. You may have heard a bit about using diet as therapy, which would make nutrition the obvious place to start, or you may have caught on to the idea that cancer is stress related, and look around for a counsellor.

If you don't know where to start, begin with your Self.

Give yourself half an hour free of interruptions and obligations.

Find four chairs and put them in a square facing each other. On the floor in front of each chair put a piece of paper on which you have identified each chair with a part of yourself:

1. Your higher self, your spirit
2. Your physical body
3. Your rational, logical thinking self
4. Your emotional, feeling self

You should not have much difficulty in seeing a distinction between your physical body and your mental activity, but some people have to work at seeing a difference between their rational, intelligent self, and their emotional, intuitive self. There are an awful lot of people who say 'I feel' when they really mean 'I think'! You might mull over that for a minute or two.

If you are uneasy about the word 'spirit' see how you feel with 'soul' or 'collective unconscious'. The idea is to find a word for that part of you that is not physical/mechanical or emotional/logical, but that is detached from all these processes. The part of you that is your own 'wise observer'. You could even call it that.

1. Start in the chair labelled Higher Self, spirit or whatever.
    Relax and close your eyes. Think about the idea that there is a part of you that is watching the rest of you. That is not tangled up with your comings and goings. A part that is detached and free. Allow yourself to feel refreshed by this idea. Try to let go of all the other aspects of yourself

and have an awareness of this wise companion that you have with you all the time.

If any special thoughts or symbols come into your head, write them down on the piece of paper.

2. Move into the chair labelled Physical Body.

Relax and close your eyes. Wander around your body. Where do you have tension? Where do you have pain? Which parts of you do you like or dislike? Are you hungry? Are you cold? How does your body feel about the way you look after it?

If any special thoughts or symbols come into your head, write them down on the paper.

Return for a moment or two to the chair for your Higher Self.

3. Move to the chair representing your logical, rational self.

What's going on here? Is your intellect being exercised in the life you lead? Are you listening to your own wisdom? What do you know and understand as distinct from what you sense and feel?

If any special thoughts and symbols come into your head, write them down on the paper.

Go back for a few moments and get in touch again with your Higher Self.

4. Sit in the chair that is identified with your emotions and feelings. What are your emotions right now? What are you feeling? Are there certain emotions you feel comfortable with and others you avoid? Do you want to cry? To laugh? To shout?

If any special thoughts or symbols come into your head, write them down on the paper.

Return for a final few moments with your Higher Self.

You can take the chairs in any order you like, but after each one return for a minute or two to the Higher Self. This means that whilst you will occupy the chairs for the body, the mind, and the emotions just once each, you will occupy the one representing your Higher Self four times in all.

In time you will find it useful to address a specific question to the various aspects of yourself, but to begin with I suggest you just try to identify clearly with the different parts and find out what's going on with each of them. See what they have to say to you.

This is a very simple exercise that you can do on your own and you can repeat it whenever you like. Always keep the pieces of paper, even if they are all blank! Date them and toss them in a box. You won't be sorry because they will make a fascinating record in years to come. Pay special attention to any images or symbols that come up and note them in your book. Later you may be able to incorporate them into affirmations or visualizations.

The first thing this exercise will do is reveal which part of you has the most to say. One patient told me,

My higher Self said all was well, even though I had cancer, everything that mattered was still quite all right. My logical, intellectual Self was full of the fact that I could fight back, that not everyone who got cancer died of it, that there was plenty I could get busy with. My physical body said it had not suffered much and it seemed to be coping very well. It was when I got to my emotions that the trouble started. What a performance! All the strength and comfort that I had felt coming from other aspects of myself was swamped in a torrent of feelings. Although three-quarters of the team were trying to reassure me, this one part was blotting out everything else and completely calling the shots.

This would be useful information to have on at least two counts. On the one hand she felt encouraged: things were not as bad as she had thought. There were parts of her staying steady, areas of herself where even having cancer was a manageable event. She found this reassuring and strengthening. On the other hand her emotions were running away with her. This was the part of her that was out of control, this was where she needed to concentrate her efforts.

The situation will differ from person to person. Another patient described the experience like this:

> My poor old body had a lot to say. I became aware that I had treated my body very badly over the years. My mind and my intellect being full of plans, schemes and new ideas had pushed my physical self to its absolute limits. I remembered with shame times when I had forced myself to continue with projects and activities when my body was spent and exhausted. My mind was having a very stimulating and entertaining time – my body was on the point of collapse.

Indeed it *had* collapsed, with a serious disease, and small wonder. Many patients admit that they have been caught up in lives so busy and competitive that their minds have been racing ahead with schemes and plans, literally dragging the poor, exhausted body behind.

Being aware of the punishing way we may have bullied our bodies in the past makes changes in diet much more meaningful. I felt I was thanking my body with appropriate and due rewards. The same was true of the relaxation exercises which I saw as a ritual acknowledgement of my past thoughtlessness and a way of repairing the damage I might have done.

Begin with a therapy that suits you.

Once you have decided which part of you most needs support or attention, choose a therapy related in some way to that area.

It is true that whatever you do will influence every part of you in the long term, but there is a pleasing sense of appropriateness in starting out like this. Once you have made the changes needed to accommodate your immediate needs you will find the space and energy to include something else. I remember a woman in her thirties, a dietitian, who had been employed for several years testing artificial sweeteners. During the course of her work she consumed large amounts of these substances while comparing their tastes in different drinks. She was quite certain that this had contributed to the development of her cancer. This, and her background in nutrition, made her keen to start her recovery programme with a disciplined and determined diet. After a few months she became interested in meditation techniques and incorporated this into her daily plan as well.

I think if a therapy feels appropriate to us, this is the perfect place to start.

As far as possible try to make balanced progress.

Look again at the model on page 36. Remind yourself that you are a spiritual and emotional being that happens to be housed in a body. Remember everything about you influences everything else.

For example, if you start with the diet, then, before trying to organize all the vitamins and minerals which are also rather body-orientated, you might find yourself a spiritual healer. When you have done this and made your visits a part of your new way of life, then maybe you might start experimenting with relaxation or meditation.

Because we are shockingly aware that cancer is manifesting itself in our physical body there is a very natural – and to a certain extent very prudent – tendency to go hammer and tongs at anything that looks remotely like a physical therapy. (I think this explains why so many people are obsessed with the diet.) There are two things that make me question whether this is entirely wise. For one thing most cancer patients are automatically given a good deal of physical therapy in hospital, so the cry for attention that is coming from the physical body may already have been acknowledged and a response made. My second anxiety concerns a tendency to pursue physical therapies of one sort or another, to the exclusion of all else. If we do this we may be ignoring cries for help from other parts of ourselves.

Ten years of working with a wide variety of physical ailments in my acupuncture clinic, and five years with cancer patients at Bristol have revealed something very clearly to me. People will struggle on without help through the most awful spiritual difficulties, they will tolerate the most punishing levels of emotional stress and intellectual frustration, and do nothing. But as soon as anything happens to their physical body they seek help. People whose suffering at emotional and spiritual levels is awesome will often hug this to themselves for years and years, and yet quite cheerfully, within a week, seek help for a stiff neck or a headache. Is this just another manifestation of the materialism of our times? No doubt it is.

There is no need to go into the reasons for why this should be the case. It doesn't take much imagination to work out what would happen if you told your boss you were wounded spiritually and needed time off work to go on a retreat. The point is, we are quick to acknowledge the manifestation of cancer on the physical body, but slow to perceive its effects on us mentally, emotionally or spiritually. Be open to this possibility and keep your programme balanced. Even if you are not aware of having cancer of the spirit or cancer of the soul, allow for the fact that you might have, and draw in therapies that will encourage healing in those areas too.

Keep adding things slowly and gradually.

See the new life that you are putting together for yourself as a tapestry. Each therapy – be it meditation, counselling, improved nutrition, acupuncture, healing, vitamin C – is another thread for you to weave into the picture. Don't try to do too many things at once or you will get into the most awful tangle. I understand only too well how urgent the situation feels when you have cancer and how frantically one wants to tear into anything that might help. Keep calm. You will create chaos and confusion if you overload yourself. Don't try in the space of a single day, or even a week, to work out how you are going to pay for counselling/persuade your doctor to prescribe vitamins/drive miles into the country to buy organically grown food. This will cause you stress and anxiety and be totally counter-productive.

Those of us bred and raised in modern capitalist society are obsessed with the idea that we must do everything in a hurry. It may be precisely this orientation to life that has contributed to our being ill. Take it easy.

Don't compare your programme with what anybody else is doing.

It should be pretty obvious that using a model of disease that says we are all sick for our own special reasons will lead to us all getting better in our own unique way. Unfortunately, even if we believe and understand this in our hearts, intuitively, as soon as we meet someone who says, 'I would have thought you would be having iscador tratment', or 'Surely you don't eat aubergines', we respond from our heads, intellectually, where we are still thinking along the old lines.

Each one of us brings into the present moment a diverse and fascinating bundle of factors that are uniquely our own. We have a certain kind of physical constitution, passed on genetically by our parents; we have a medical history of hay-fever or stomach ulcers; we may work in an asbestos factory or we may not have to work at all; we may be loved, valued and cherished by the world or we may be lonely, ignored and abandoned; we may be life-long vegetarians or we may eat only convenience, junk foods, we may smoke, be on the Pill, live near a leaky nuclear power station – the list goes on and on. Remind yourself of this if someone puts pressure on you to conform to what they think you should be doing.

When people say 'If I were you' they mean precisely that. They are telling you what they would do, or what they are already doing. Hopefully they are doing what is right for them, but it may never be a part of your master plan. When we compare ourselves with other people we often stir up feelings of rivalry. This is a pattern of behaviour learned at school and in the cut and thrust of the business world, but it is inappropriate now. Healing yourself of cancer is not a competition where people come in first, second or third.

Holistic cancer control is a process, not an event.

This way of dealing with disease is not something you do for a while and then stop, like having an operation or a course of radiotherapy treatment.

I would love to be able to say that if you follow a detailed set of instructions for a fixed length of time then the whole cancer business will be behind you. That it will become a past event, something you did in the 1980s that is over and done with. Unfortunately the chances are that it will not be like that. I became very excited at the apparent success of my efforts to heal myself, rushed back into work far too soon, and promptly grew another lump. I have met countless people who, following surgery, radiotherapy or chemotherapy, were declared quite well again, but were back in hospital within the year. Experience shows us that many people have several encounters with cancer. It would be asking a lot for us to get this right first time. Cancer is such a puzzling disease. A London consultant told me that he had seen examples of patients in whom one cancer lump was getting smaller, and another getting bigger, at the same time. This is just another thing that points us back to the fact that cancer is an idiosyncratic disease with a sometimes most erratic course. It is not always easy to know when we have it and when we don't, when we are getting better and when we aren't.

Anyway, we might be missing the point. For many people illness has meaning. They see it as part of their growth process and consequently they do not feel it is a disaster that must be annihilated at once. Even if you don't feel like this, don't imagine that this kind of self-help programme is as simple and straightforward as taking antibiotics for the prescribed length of time. If you don't make the sort of dramatic progress you expect, don't feel that you have failed, or that you didn't try hard enough. The changes that you are working towards will not happen cataclysmically, they will unfold. Remember, a process, not an event.

Now ask yourself what you are hoping to achieve.

Most people's primary goal is to get rid of their cancer. This is true for most patients, but it is a goal largely based on the belief that anything else spells death and disaster. Allow yourself to open up your hopes and expectations a bit, don't be too rigid and fixed about your goals. If you are going to judge your progress only against what your doctor tells you or what the hospital says, you may make life unnecessarily difficult and disappointing for yourself.

I thought for a long time that while I could still be diagnosed as a cancer patient by way of the usual clinical signs, then I would still be 'sick'. I could not imagine leading a healthy, happy life and still having cancer. Yes, I did say healthy. I have a tumour in my left breast that has stubbornly resisted all my marvellous strategies for getting rid of it completely for more than three years. Initially there was a period of intense anxiety when the hospital were asking me to go for check-ups every three weeks on the basis that it would spread all over the place in no time at all. I managed to resist treatment during this time and started a revised self-help programme. I grew fitter and stronger and the lump grew smaller. I now go every six months and nobody knows quite what to make of it. In the meantime I am running around having a lovely life, a lot less scared and inconvenienced by having a lump in my breast than many of my friends are by a life of constantly checking theirs.

When I first had the cancer diagnosed one of the staff nurses

Possible parts of a Holistic therapy

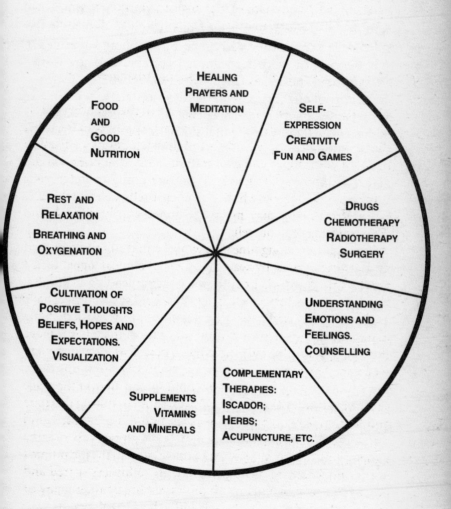

FOOD AND GOOD NUTRITION

HEALING PRAYERS AND MEDITATION

SELF-EXPRESSION CREATIVITY FUN AND GAMES

REST AND RELAXATION BREATHING AND OXYGENATION

DRUGS CHEMOTHERAPY RADIOTHERAPY SURGERY

CULTIVATION OF POSITIVE THOUGHTS BELIEFS, HOPES AND EXPECTATIONS. VISUALIZATION

UNDERSTANDING EMOTIONS AND FEELINGS. COUNSELLING

SUPPLEMENTS VITAMINS AND MINERALS

COMPLEMENTARY THERAPIES: ISCADOR; HERBS; ACUPUNCTURE, ETC.

told me I would just have to learn to live with it. I would have taken more kindly to this suggestion if I had thought such a thing was possible. Now I know that it is.

Many times I hear from patients who go back to hospital feeling well and happy only to be told that X-rays and blood tests show sinister signs. I am well aware that nothing can quite equal the sense of achievement that accompanies the knowledge that the cancer has gone, but we should not suggest that the person who has achieved comfort and joy in the presence of cancer has failed. Most of us would opt for a shorter life of quality if the alternative was to buy extra time at the expense of suffering. This being so, a programme that so enhances the quality of life that the patient no longer feels ill, (or fits the clinical signs) should surely be deemed a success.

Assess your needs.

Imagine that this diagram is showing a cake that is made up of eight marked slices. Now think of these eight sections as being ingredients you need to make the cake. Dr Hywell Williams, currently working at Charing Cross Hospital, said in a recent interview, he thought that doctors could help with about a third of the sick person's needs ('and that's being generous') while the rest of their healing would come from their own resources.

Write in your book which of these parts of the whole do you have most of, and which are in short supply. This simple exercise will show you very clearly that you should not take too much notice of what other people are doing. Their shopping list will be different from yours.

It will also show you that you are well on the way to supplying the requirements of some of these ingredients. You can establish this more clearly if you fill out some of the sections with extra things that might be available to you. Things like enrolling in a yoga class, joining a choir, taking a course in wholefood cookery and so on. Remember this is only a model for you to play around with. Its value lies in reminding us to keep broadening our base and widening our perspectives. Neither Bristol, nor this book, could contain all the healing possibilities available to us.

Yesterday I was talking to a woman at Bristol who said that she had brought her sister with her, and explained that the cancer had brought the two of them together again after years of estrangement. 'You see,' she said, 'it's not all bad!' Indeed it is not and the next exercise is to do with this phenomenon.

Make a list of advantages of having cancer.

For some people this is a shocking idea and they resent it very much. You may feel that you simply cannot think of anything good at all about being ill. Even if you can the chances are that you won't want to admit to it. If you find all this too painful, skip it and come back to it another time.

Think of these things as secondary gains or unexpected spin-offs of the situation. The story of the lady reunited with her sister is an example of what you might put down, but not all secondary gains are going to sound quite so laudable. Once you get going you might be surprised at what you come up with, but don't suppress anything. I was almost frightened at the benefits I found myself admitting to, but this information was to prove very useful to me later. My list consisted of things like:

My husband doesn't shout at me any more.

People are kind and loving to me.

I am the centre of attention.

These confessions didn't make me feel very wonderful about myself but they were most revealing. I was getting a glimpse of a side of myself that had been hidden from me up until that time. I often hear patients say things like, 'Well, at least this gives me the excuse to go for early redundancy', or 'I never wanted to emigrate to Australia anyway'.

The important thing about recognizing our secondary gains

is that they represent needs and wishes that we have not been able to fulfil until now. If we do not find other ways of achieving what we want in this life the cancer may become so useful to us that we need to hang on to it. Or, having got rid of it, get it again. Cancer is a powerful weapon with which we can threaten the world around us. I only have to say I feel a bit run-down and tired, and I don't know why but I haven't been feeling myself lately, to bring my family to its knees. Fortunately for all of us I have acquired other ways of getting a bit of help with the washing up, but I rest my case.

This leads us to look at why some people have such difficulty in getting what they want out of life.

Is your personality working for you or against you? Do you have a cancer personality?

This question may strike you as being rather ridiculous if you are suffering from mesothelioma brought on by asbestos poisoning, but think again. You can't do anything about your past exposure to asbestos, but you can change your present behaviour patterns, and these behaviour patterns may be critically important. We know that not everyone exposed to a known carcinogen develops cancer. We know that other factors may be tipping the balance between fighting off disease and succumbing to it. One of these factors is to do with how we behave.

Dr David Kissen, a Scottish physician researching into lung cancer in men, established that those among the male, smoking, population who developed cancer had no adequate outlet for their emotions. Research in America has suggested that 'bitchy' women with breast cancer have the best prognosis.

Over the years many different people working with cancer patients have observed in them certain characteristics that seem to emerge with great frequency. I have put together both the qualities that we have been most struck by at Bristol and

the characteristics most often remarked upon by other therapists.

1. Cancer patients are often do-gooders. They are kind, nice
   people, often employed in the 'caring professions', and
   looking for ways of helping others.
2. They are uncomfortable about expressing negative
   emotions, particularly in their own defence. They find it
   hard to say 'no'.
3. They have a low self-image.

If we look closely at these characteristic tendencies we see a
picture emerging. Some people have been trained from
childhood to earn affection as a reward for good deeds. This
establishes the idea that one is not loved for oneself, only for
what one does. Naturally this makes it very hard to say 'no' –
to stop being nice and good for a while – because that might
lead to a withdrawal of affection from the world. Continuing
to perform in a certain way, even when you don't want to, can
lead to high levels of frustration. But there is no outlet
available for a person who thinks so little of themselves that
they dare not stop 'buying' affection and approval. They may
be fed up and furious inside, but still smiling and saying 'yes'
on the outside.

Elsewhere I have described a patient who thought so little of
herself that she could not even imagine herself well as part of a
visualization exercise. It is not impossible that some of us feel
so miserable about ourselves we feel we deserve to die. Cancer
is one way of doing it.

If you are one of the people for whom none of this has any
meaning it might interest you to know that every week at
Bristol this description of the so-called 'cancer personality'
brings tears of recognition to the eyes of many of our patients.

It is sometimes quite a struggle for people to accept the idea
that they have the right to behave in any other way. Their
knowledge of life may have led them to associate assertiveness
with aggression. It is possible that the only expression of

negative feeling they ever experienced as children was always accompanied by violence. In such circumstances even something as harmless as saying 'no' becomes charged with meaning. But if we can't say 'no' at a behavioural level, maybe we can't do it at a physical level either.

I have often thought how the performance of a person reflecting all these characteristics resembles what is happening in the body of a cancer patient. When we say 'no' to a request or an event that is presenting itself to us in life we are marking our boundaries. We are saying, 'I will accept this, but I won't accept that.' We are protecting ourselves against things that we sense are not in our interests, things that will exhaust us or do us harm. This is what a healthy person does when faced with the challenge of cancer cells. The body's system of self-defence recognizes a threat and says 'no'. Since this is precisely the state of affairs that we are trying to activate in our bodies, it may be useful to look at ways in which we can do the same thing in other areas of our existence.

Watch out for saboteurs.

There are many people who say that cancer brought them closer to husbands, wives, children, friends and so on. They talk of people rallying around and friendships firming up and becoming stronger. Unfortunately it is not always like that.

There are always going to be people around who hinder rather than help. Just when you want a bit of support and encouragement someone comes along and tells you they knew a woman who had been a yoga teacher for ten years, but all that breathing and meditation didn't stop her dying of cancer. It is too depressing to list the ways in which friends, neighbours and family can undermine the fragile structure of our hopes and plans. But the fact is that they do. This is not likely to be intentional and you can often deflect and discourage it by saying, 'Oh please don't say that, I'm trying to be positive.' In this way you are pointing out quite gently that you find this person's attitude depressing and you are giving them the opportunity to change it. What you do next, if they persist in depressing you, is a very important issue.

One of the reasons we encourage patients who come to Bristol to bring a friend or member of their family with them is to ensure that they will have support from at least one other person. However, not everyone finds the environment encouraging. For some people just watching the pursuit of this kind of holistic approach to self-healing can be a difficult challenge.

If you yourself do not have cancer and have no inducement or inclination to look critically at your life and ways in which you can improve it, it can be uncomfortable to be close to someone who is doing precisely that. Sometimes patients find that as they grow and change the people around them start to resent this and tensions develop. Cracks may open in relationships that could even lead to break-ups. These cracks have always been there, but the pressure of the cancer crisis may cause them to widen. If this is the case you may find, to your sorrow, that people in close relationships are sabotaging you in ways that are hard to stop. This would be something to talk through with a counsellor if possible. Otherwise one must practise avoidance of some sort. Naturally, physical avoidance is not always possible, but it is possible to avoid looking for support from people who are not capable of giving it.

This sounds pretty obvious, but it is sometimes hard to do. I wasted a lot of time and strength trying to wrestle understanding and approval from people who had given it to me in the past, but who were not prepared to continue doing so. We are often so accustomed to leaning on some people that we imagine we cannot do without them. Struggling to make them change may bring us nothing but frustration and disappointment. If we see our attempts to gain approval and support as hangovers from the past that are no longer necessary, we shall free ourselves of some painful attachments. The more we continue to take responsibility for our lives and our healing, the less we shall need to seek from other people.

If support is hard to come by and you feel isolated and lonely, take heart. It was Carl Jung in *Modern Man in Search of a Soul* who said: 'It is, moreover, only in the state of complete abandonment and loneliness that we experience the helpful powers of our own natures.'

If that sounds too much like 'making the best of it', remember that even the people who are cosily supported by a wide circle of supporters may suffer from sabotage. In fact, often our worst enemy is our own internal saboteur. (In this respect our own natures may not be altogether helpful.) We all have a person lurking inside us ready to put us down. The voice that murmurs 'You'll never manage to do that, you're too fat/too thin/too stupid/too old/too poor/too ill/too late . . .'. Remember him? Some of us have given the internal saboteur a lot of strength over the years by listening to all this negative whispering and we may be dealing with a very well-developed sub-personality that can give us a lot of trouble. The first thing to do is to recognize that the saboteur exists, and not just in us, but in everybody. This will help us deal with negativity and depression coming from other people – it is not coming from the part of that person that loves us and wants to help, it is coming from their saboteur. The second thing is not to take it seriously.

As soon as we start arguing or reacting to the saboteur we give him power. The only way to be free of the insidious destructiveness of this side of ourselves is to ignore it. When the negative thoughts come we should observe in a detached way that the saboteur is having a go again, and ignore both him and what he says. If possible, laugh. Never reward your saboteur with internal arguments or discussions because he will *always* win.

If you wake up one morning feeling low and the saboteur says, 'They're very nice those people at Bristol, but they don't really know what they're talking about', the best reaction is to say firmly to oneself, 'I'm just going through a bad patch, this will pass' and try to let it go at that. If you respond with, 'Oh yes they do know, they are all clever and qualified', then expect something like, 'If they are that clever and qualified why isn't everyone doing what they say? Why don't their methods work every time? Why don't they teach visualization in hospital?' You will never win an argument with your internal saboteur.

One of the most enjoyable sessions for me at Bristol is to get together with a group of patients and talk about the internal saboteur. As everyone contributes their own particular version of what that miserable little voice has to say, we all quickly see that we have a lot in common. Eventually as the phrases get repeated over and over again, we see them for the stereotypes they are, and after a while it is impossible not to laugh.

Get all the help you can.

This is a good moment to introduce the **Bach Flower Remedies**. When we are trying to find the strength and equanimity to handle a rising tide of fear, negativity and emotion in general it is comforting to know we can be helped by taking a few drops of flower essences. Not every inch of ground is bought at the price of effort and struggle. These remedies are simple, safe, easy ways of helping ourselves.

I am grateful to my friends at Dr Bach's home in Sotwell for giving me permission to reprint here the contents of their introductory leaflet. This gives a brief explanation of the history of the remedies and the way in which they work, which is basically through our emotions and feelings. One of the most appealing aspects of these remedies is that they can be given to everyone who is being affected by the cancer crisis, not just the patient. I remember a time in my home when the entire family was on mimulus (for fear) and star of Bethlehem (for shock), while I was taking olive (for exhaustion) and vervain (for over-enthusiasm) as well. Thank goodness the remedies are cheap.

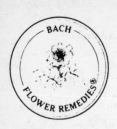
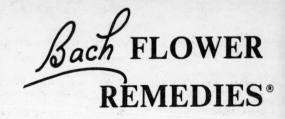

Bach FLOWER REMEDIES®

The simple and natural method of establishing complete equilibrium and harmony through the personality by means of wild flowers discovered by:
Edward Bach, M.B., B.S., M.R.C.S., L.R.C.P., D.P.H.

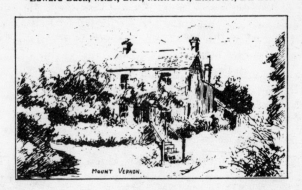

MOUNT VERNON.

All enquiries to: **BACH FLOWER REMEDIES LTD., DR. E. BACH CENTRE, MOUNT VERNON, SOTWELL, WALLINGFORD, OXON. OX10 0PZ, ENGLAND** where Dr. Bach lived and worked and in the surrounding fields and hedgerows discovered his healing flowers. The very same wild flower locations are used to this day in the preparation of the Flower Remedies by the present custodians, who are dedicated by legacy, to maintain the simple method and use of the Remedies as intended by Dr. Bach, and so faithfully carried out subsequent to the doctor's passing by the late Nora Weeks.

The 38 Remedies cover every negative state of mind known to man, and will (in keeping with Dr. Bach's express wish) remain a complete entity. Therefore no claimed 'extensions', 'furtherance' or prepared facsimile of the Bach Remedies hold any association with the Bach Centre whatsoever.

OFFICIAL OVERSEAS DISTRIBUTORS:

U.S.A./Canada: Ellon (Bach U.S.A.) Inc., P.O. Box 320, Woodmere, N.Y. 11598 U.S.A. (Tel. 516 825 2229).

Germany/Austria/Switzerland: M. Scheffer Hp., (Bach Centre German Office), Eppendorfer Landstr. 32, 2000 Hamburg 20, W. Germany. (Tel. 040 464624).

Australia: Nonesuch Botanicals Pty. Ltd., P.O. Box 68, Mt. Evelyn, Vic. 3796, Australia. (Tel. (03) 762 8577).
　　　　　Martin & Pleasance Wholesale Pty. Ltd., P.O. Box 4, Collingwood, Vic. 3066, Australia. (Tel. 419 9733).

Holland/Belgium: Holland Pharma, Postbus 37, 7240 AA Lochem, Holland. (Tel. 05730-2884)

Denmark: Camet   Murervej 16, 6700 Esbjerg, Denmark. (Tel. 05-155444).

AT A GLANCE REFERENCE TO THE BACH REMEDIES

(see price list for further reading material)

1. **Agrimony.** Those who suffer considerable inner torture which they try to dissemble behind a facade of cheerfulness.

2. **Aspen.** Apprehension — the feeling that something dreadful is going to happen without knowing why.

3. **Beech.** Critical and intolerant of others. Arrogant.

4. **Centaury.** Weakness of will; those who let themselves be exploited or imposed upon — become subservient; difficulty in saying 'no'. Human doormat.

5. **Cerato.** Those who doubt their own judgement, seeks advice of others. Often influenced and misguided.

6. **Cherry Plum.** Uncontrolled — irrational thoughts.

7. **Chestnut Bud.** Refusal to learn by experience; continually repeating the same mistakes.

8. **Chicory.** The over-possessive, demands respect or attention (selfishness), likes others to conform to their standards. Makes martyr of oneself.

9. **Clematis.** Indifferent, inattentive, dreamy, absent-minded. Mental escapist from reality.

10. **Crab Apple.** Cleanser. Feels unclean or ashamed of ailments. Self disgust/hatred. House proud.

11. **Elm.** Temporarily overcome by inadequacy or responsibility. Normally very capable.

12. **Gentian.** Despondent. Easily discouraged and dejected.

13. **Gorse.** Pessimistic — 'Oh what's the use'. Defeatism.

14. **Heather.** People who are obsessed with their own troubles and experiences. Talkative 'bores' — poor listeners.

15. **Holly.** For those who are jealous, envious, revengeful and suspicious. For those who hate.

16. **Honeysuckle.** For those with nostalgia and who constantly dwell in the past. Home-sickness.

17. **Hornbeam.** 'Monday morning' feeling but once started, task usually fulfilled. Procrastination.

18. **Impatiens.** Impatience, irritability.

19. **Larch.** Despondency due to lack of self-confidence; expectation of failure, so fails to make the attempt. Feels inferior, yet has the ability.

20. **Mimulus.** Fear of *known* things. Shyness, timidity.

21. **Mustard.** 'Dark cloud' that descends for no known reason which can lift just as suddenly making one downcast, saddened and low.

22. **Oak.** Brave determined types. Struggles on in illness and against adversity despite setbacks. Plodders.

23. **Olive.** Drained of energy — everything an effort. Fatigued.

24. **Pine.** Feelings of guilt. Blames self for mistakes of other. Feels unworthy.

25. **Red Chestnut.** Over care and excessive concern for others, especially those held dear.

26. **Rock Rose.** Alarmed, scared, panicky, full of trepidation.

27. **Rock Water.** For those who are hard on themselves — often overwork. Rigid minded, self denying.

28. **Scleranthus.** Uncertainty/indecision/vacillation. Fluctuating moods.

29. **Star of Bethlehem.** For all the effects of serious news, or fright following an accident, etc.

30. **Sweet Chestnut.** Absolute dejection.

31. **Vervain.** Over-enthusiasm, over effort; straining. Fanatical and highly-strung. Incensed and frustrated by injustices.

32. **Vine.** Dominating / inflexible / ambitious / tyrannical/autocratic. Arrogant pride. Considered to be good leaders.

33. **Walnut.** Protection remedy from powerful influences, and helps adjustment to any transition or change, e.g. puberty, menopause, divorce, new surroundings.

34. **Water Violet.** Proud, reserved, sedate types, sometimes 'superior'. Little emotional involvement but reliable/dependable.

35. **White Chestnut.** Persistent unwanted thoughts. Pre-occupation with some worry or episode. Mental arguments.

36. **Wild Oat.** Helps determine one's intended path in life.

37. **Wild Rose.** Resignation, apathy. Drifters who accept their lot, making little effort for improvement — lacks ambition.

38. **Willow.** Resentment and bitterness with 'not fair' and 'poor me' attitude.

39. **RESCUE REMEDY.** A combination of Cherry Plum, Clematis, Impatiens, Rock Rose, Star of Bethlehem. All purpose emergency composite for effects of anguish, examinations, going to the dentist, etc. Comforting, calming and reassuring to those distressed by startling experiences.

THE BACH SYSTEM

The Remedies used are all prepared from the flowers of wild plants, bushes and trees, and none of them is harmful or habit-forming.

They are used, **not directly,** for physical complaints, but for the sufferer's worry, apprehension, hopelessness, irritability, etc., because these states of mind or moods not only hinder recovery of health and retard convalescence, but are generally accepted as primary causes of sickness and disease.

A long-continued worry or fear, as is well-known, will deplete the individual's vitality; he will feel out of sorts, below par, not himself and the body then loses its natural resistance. As peace and harmony is achieved, unity returns to mind and body, closing the circuit as it were and allowing the Life Force to flow freely again, thus providing the body its chance to produce its own **natural** healing.

This system and the Remedies were discovered by a doctor who had practised for over 20 years in London as a Harley Street consultant, bacteriologist and homoeopath. The late Edward Bach, M.B., B.S., M.R.C.S., L.R.C.P., D.P.H., gave up his lucrative practice in 1930 to devote his full time to seek energies in the plant world which would restore vitality to the sick, so that the sufferer himself would be able to overcome his worry, his apprehension, etc., and so assist in his own healing.

Dr. Bach developed great sensitivity both in mind and body. If he held his hand over a flowering plant, or the flower in the palm of his hand, he could sense in himself the properties of that flower.

Before finding a particular flower, he would suffer in himself, and very acutely, the negative state of mind for which that flower was needed and, at the same time, he was priviledged, as he said, to suffer from some physical complaint. Then he would wander about the fields and lanes until he was 'led' to find the flowers which would immediately restore his serenity and peace of mind, and within a few hours the physical complaint would also be healed.

In this way he found 38 flowers to cover all known negative states of mind from which mankind can suffer, categorizing them in seven headings. Those for apprehension. For uncertainty and indecision. For loneliness. For insufficient interest in present circumstances. For over-sensitiveness to ideas and influence. For despondency and despair. For over-care for the welfare of others.

As the Bach Remedies are benign in their action and can result in no unpleasant reactions, they can be taken by anyone. Stock Concentrate Remedies will keep indefinitely — a 10ml size concentrate bottle will provide sufficient to make approx. 60 treatment bottles. More than one Remedy can be taken at the same time — 2 drops of each chosen Remedy in a cup of water and sipped at intervals, or in a 30ml (1 fl.oz.) bottle filled with spring water (*this represents a treatment bottle*) from which 4 drops are taken directly on the tongue at least 4 times a day.

Literature and issued instructions are self-explanatory, making it quite simple for sufferers to help themselves and others. If further advice is then required a brief word picture is needed of a person's personality, temperament, general outlook, worries, etc., and reasons for same if any. Any great disappointment or upset which might have left its mark, and what effect it has had on your thoughts, actions, outlook and so on.

Please remember — consider the person's attitude of mind, feelings, worries, indecision, timidity, vexations, resentment, possessiveness, hopelessness, lethargy, hatred, overpowering or demanding nature, intolerance, tenseness, etc., and most essentially the reason 'why' there is apprehension, worry and fear, for only then will the correct remedy(s) be determined — physical conditions are only considered as a guide to the person's state of suffering and its subsequent effect on the sufferer's outlook.

It is up to the person to take medical advice if necessary.

Consultation and advice freely given.

The 'RESCUE REMEDY' (Liquid or Cream)

Dr. Bach combined five specific Remedies from the 38 to formulate an emergency composite that he chose to call 'Rescue Remedy'. He saved a fisherman's life in 1930 with this preparation.

Its purpose is to comfort/reassure and calm those who have received serious news, severe upset, startling experiences consequently falling into a numbed, bemused state of mind.

To nullify the sufferer's anguish is of the utmost importance in helping the natural healing process of one's being to proceed without hindrance, so the 'Rescue Remedy' is invaluable to keep at hand for immediate use until the arrival of the doctor if necessary. It does not take the place of medical attention.

'Rescue Remedy' is taken orally (4 drops in water), but can also be applied externally either in liquid or cream form — see instruction leaflet. **Animals and plants can also benefit from this treatment.**

Since we always encourage people who come to Bristol to bring a friend or a relative with them as well we have the opportunity of introducing a wide circle of the patient's family to these remedies. This can only be good. The remedies help everyone involved to cope with the challenge that the cancer crisis presents to them.

When you read the list of characteristics relating to the remedies there is a tendency to imagine you need them all! This is quite understandable because the remedies relate to states of mind that we are all likely to have experienced at some time or another. There is nothing wrong with this. What we are looking for is whether we have a tendency to respond to our experience of the world with one particular reaction more than any other. Is there a particular feeling that predominates? Sometimes one special remedy appeals to us straight away as being just the right one for us, but it would not be unusual or inappropriate to take several remedies at once if the situation demanded it.

I have used these remedies for years. For my patients in my acupuncture practice, for my friends and for my family, and of course they have been used at Bristol ever since we began. I have never ceased to be awed and amazed at how effective they are. I admit I am the sort of person who wants to believe in such things, but perhaps a more impressive testimonial would come from my husband whose initial cynicism led him to suggest, 'There are fairies at the bottom of the bottle I suppose. . . ?' He is now as dedicated a devotee as I am – but only after a long course of vine.

When making enquiries about these remedies please remember to enclose a stamped addressed envelope. The dedicated service offered by the group of people who work from Mount Sotwell is truly amazing. The prices are kept as low as possible and remedies are almost always received by return of post.

Under this question of getting help something must also be said about *asking* for help. You will get more support if you can identify your needs clearly and make them known. If you recognize in yourself some of the characteristics of the 'cancer personality' you may find it easier to give help than to receive it. This might mean that you are a bit difficult to reach, and friends who would like to do something for you may feel cut off from you. You may be the sort of person who gives the impression of being so self-sufficient and well organized that offers of help are almost an intrusion. You can break through all this by simply asking for help directly, and being very specific about what help you want. If you find it easier, then wait for the moment when someone next says to you 'There must be something I can do', and leap in with, 'Yes, there is.' It may come as a surprise to people to hear that you would like them to look after the children for half an hour so you can have a bit of peace and quiet for a meditation, or do your ironing for you while you visit your healer. They may have had it in mind to pass a cool hand across your fevered brow and arrange a few flowers, but they will get far more satisfaction from doing something that you really want.

Since the restrictions of the diet often impose limitations on one's social life – at least for a while – then you could ask your friends to help by cooking you a meal from time to time. There are lots of benefits to be had from doing this. You get a night out and a bit of welcome entertainment for a start. And more than likely a delicious and imaginative meal. When people are cooking for a dinner party or special occasion, they will go to a lot more trouble than you do on an average day. They are going to eat this food with you so they have their own interests at heart as well as yours. All things considered they are likely to put up a good show, and this may help to inspire you and give you a few good ideas about cooking for yourself. Get your friends to read the chapter on nutrition in this book or Sadhya Rippon's recipe book. You will be doing them a favour as well as yourself.

Whatever you are doing, give it your attention and awareness.

In some respects this is just another way of saying 'don't do everything at once', but there is a little more to it than that. If we are trying to do too much we end up by operating a sort of automatic pilot. We get through a chain of activities in a repetitive and mindless way and can hardly remember whether we have done something or not. This kind of rush is not conducive to healing. We should pause for a moment before eating our food and bring an intention and an awareness to the activity of eating it. Better still would be to allow a moment to give thanks for it, to bless it. Every time I say 'Bless this food to my use and my self to Thy service' I bring my attention back from the clatter of everyday existence and focus for a moment on something else.

This is similar to the idea of bringing the mind back to concentrating on the breath during relaxation. We can do this when we are taking vitamins or shopping for food. Instead of planning the next thing we are going to do, where we are going after we've seen the healer, we should try to live in the moment, and be conscious of what we are doing at that particular time. If our therapies start running away with us and we start reacting instead of acting we have begun to lose control.

You can never fail.

When medicine just consists of treatment to physical symptoms it makes sense to talk of it in terms of success and failure. But when we set out to heal ourselves the situation is different. We embark on a journey towards wholeness which means that every step we take is another step towards understanding; every step brings us nearer to enlightenment. We may or we may not subdue the sickness in our physical body and alter its behaviour according to our wishes; we may rejoice in achieving that or let go of it as an objective. In the end we shall be journeying for its own sake, not to reach a specific destination. All travellers always arrive eventually.

THE BROADER PERSPECTIVE

'He who saves the life of a single soul, saves the whole world.' *The Talmud.*

I am acutely aware as I write this book that the medical model is getting bigger and bigger. We have moved outwards from the narrow perspective of looking only at the cancer cells and the way they behave, towards a view of the patient as a whole and the way he himself behaves in the environment in which he lives.

I am talking about cancer and the meaning of illness in a way that might make sense to a mature, fairly intelligent adult. Ringing in my ears is the question I am always asked, 'But what about children?'

Does it make sense to see disease as 'an opportunity for change' in the life of a tiny infant? Can one sensibly talk about 'the cancer personality' in relation to a two-year old with leukaemia? No, I don't think you can. But that does not mean that there is no value or purpose in looking at these questions in a broader context.

Cancer in children presents us with the challenge of looking at the kind of environment in which these children are raised. I have a close friend whose daughter is recovering from Hodgkins' disease. She and her husband have talked to me about their feelings that they may have been in part responsible for this. They saw, on reflection, that they had cut themselves off from this child by their intense involvement with their own lives: the development of their own careers; the need to put her into boarding school, and so on. They chose to look at the problem in the broad context of their family life and saw the disease as a way that their child could use to draw them all closer together again.

By saying this I am most emphatically not saying that all parents are responsible for their children's diseases. I have experienced at first hand the terrible sense of guilt that accompanies any threat to the well-being of one's children. I found my third child, aged three months, blue in her cot, inert and not breathing. A frantic race to the hospital and her partial restoration in an oxygen tent with the warning 'we have a very sick child on our hands – has she been christened?' that left me hysterical with guilt. I discovered for myself something that is well known to all who nurse or administer to sick children, that parents always feel guilty and ashamed when their children are ill. They may need to be absolved from this. The very last thing they need is someone suggesting that it is indeed their fault.

There is no reason why it should be the parents' fault, but I think we should not deny the possibility that it might be. Neither should we close our eyes to the possibility that it might be our collective fault, that society has a responsibility towards its children.

Some children are raised in an inhospitable emotional environment that they find hard to bear. Why should this not act as a stress factor, potentially damaging to their immune system, in the same way as we acknowledge that this might be so of an adult? It is not necessarily the case, but we should allow for the fact that it might be. We may not be able to sew this up as neatly as we would like. There may be circumstances where we incline to the view that 'the parents have eaten sour grapes and the children's teeth are set on edge'. But at other times we are reminded of Jesus's rebuke to his disciples when they suggested that disease was always a legacy of sin. 'Neither this man did sin, nor his parents' . . . was his unequivocal response to that suggestion.

We should not be afraid of looking into these problems, neither should we prejudge the answer. The question is one of responsibility, not guilt.

I know another couple, much younger, whose first baby

A Broader Holistic Model of Man

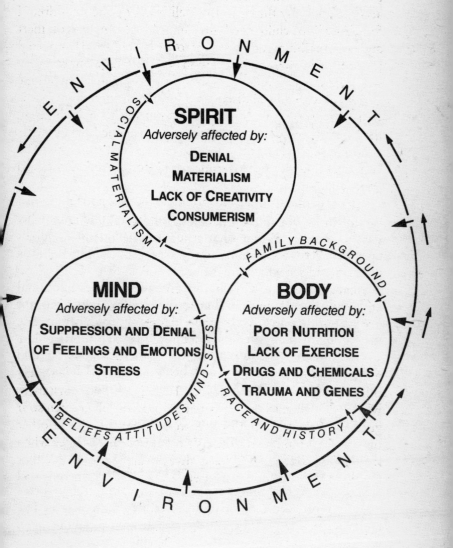

showed signs of cancer within months of being born. I watched them as they nursed this little soul tenderly and lovingly while a huge tumour took over a large part of his brain. Gradually his eyes glazed over, he didn't move about much, his feeding became slow and laboured, and it became quite clear to us all that he was going to die. He took a very long time to die. I never for one moment felt that his parents were responsible for any of this. I saw this baby as a victim of what some people would call 'original sin' or what others would call 'environmental pollution'. Watching and witnessing his serene progress I could also see how some people would fit this event into a view of the universe that holds with reincarnation and karmic destiny.

The model on page 195 shows how many factors may be influencing our health and wellbeing. While it is true we can effect some direct degree of control over some of these, it is very obvious we can do little about others. I think it would be wise to do for children what adults can do for themselves – take a broad overview of as many aspects of the child's life as possible and see which areas need the most help. Then we do what we can. It is always hard to see the difference between guilt and responsibility in this kind of context, but of course there is a difference. Perhaps we can only really learn about prevention through direct experience of the crisis itself.

The thought of children with cancer raises more sharply than anything the idea of people being 'victims' of cancer. We cannot comfortably hold a child responsible for his life in quite the way we can an adult. If it emerges quite clearly that a child has been overworked and undernourished it is usually true that he has had little, if any, control over these areas of his life. It requires someone else to take responsibility for these things and start to change them on the child's behalf.

We now know that people suffering from tuberculosis require more than an assault on the disease itself. The mortality rate from tuberculosis was dropping rapidly years before the discovery of the TB bacillus, in response to environmental improvements. In their book *The Healing Arts*

Kaptchuk and Croucher have this to say about drug treatment in relation to tuberculosis.

> These drugs can only cure when the environment is properly administered; they have not affected the incidence of TB in those countries where living conditions are similar to those of nineteenth-century Britain. Most of the other dreaded infectious diseases of the last century disappeared because of life-style and environmental changes as did leprosy and bubonic plague in earlier centuries.

This does not mean that one should not acknowledge the role played by drugs and antibiotics: it means one should acknowledge that other factors may also play a very important role. It looks very likely that cancer will prove to have a similar history to tuberculosis. The shift from the disease to the environment is already taking place. It is strange that it should have taken so long. Even Louis Pasteur, who did more than anyone to focus attention on the identification of the germs that cause disease, is reputed to have said at the end of his life that the microbes were less important than the soil in which they grew. When Josef Issels talks about the cancer 'milieu' I think we are witnessing the same shift, and we should welcome it.

Although the whole thrust and tenor of this book is about people taking responsibility for their disease and doing things to help themselves, nevertheless it must be said that there is a sense in which we are all victims.

Remember the good old days when it was 'immoral or illegal or it made you fat'? Well, these days it gives you cancer. The list of substances, activities, performances and events that have been linked to cancer in some way or another is now so vast it has led to a great deal of confusion and cynicism. People are so thoroughly fed up with being warned against E-numbers in processed food and nitrates in fresh food they declare that if they listened to every warning they heard then they would never eat at all. One cannot but have a certain sympathy for this.

I know that there are days when I feel a bit overwhelmed by the number of things I cannot control. Since the Chernobyl disaster there has been much talk of radiation from such apparent innocent sources as the colour television set. This was something that I was made aware of many years ago and I fixed up my living room so that I could watch the television reflected in a mirror. Just when I was thinking how clever I was being someone came along and told me that, although I might be avoiding the rays from my own television, how did I know I wasn't picking up the radiation from the television next door? I had no idea such a thing was possible and now I had something else to worry about. For those of us lucky enough to live in houses well detached from our neighbours this may not be a problem, but what about terraces? What about flats?

I often meet cancer patients who have made the most heroic and successful effort to give up smoking, but just as they are giving themselves a congratulatory pat on the back for this they read an article about the harmful effects of 'secondary' smoking. They then have to face the fact that they are working in an open office where everyone else is puffing away like a chimney. It is hard not to feel helpless and demoralized in these circumstances.

The harsh reality is that, even if we do everything in our power to help ourselves, cancer patients are vulnerable in a broader context, a context over which they have very little control.

It was Karl Marx who said, 'The philosophers have only interpreted the world, the point, however, is to change it.' In this respect I agree with him entirely. No book that interests itself with cancer in an individual can sensibly ignore cancer in the community. By the same token we cannot meaningfully attempt to heal ourselves without trying to heal our environment as well.

Every time we ask for organically grown vegetables at the local shops we are paving the way for change. Farmers will continue to use high-yield chemical production methods in defiance of a million warning words written in medical journals and scientific reports. But they will change their tune overnight in response to market forces. As soon as it is worth their while, in their economic interests, they will start to farm with care and boastfully advertise the fact that they do. This is already beginning to happen. I often pass small farms with proud placards bearing assertions to the effect that 'these fields have been organically grown for 5 years'. The message is beginning to get home.

In the same way we should have the courage to petition for the kind of water we want to drink. Even if we can be reasonably sure that our reservoirs are not filling up with chemicals washed off the fields, are we at all sure what is being added to our water at the processing plants? If we don't want to be 'fluorided' we must take the trouble to say so, to write to our MP, ask questions, get involved. Not everyone can afford to buy bottled water, and anyway why should we?

It is only public awareness that will bring about these changes. The petroleum companies are not going to remove the lead from petrol that adds that extra edge to our air pollution unless we insist that they do. There are countries which insist on lead-free petrol; we should do the same.

We cannot afford to go down in a welter of helpless self-pity about these things. The recent anxiety over additives has led to certain supermarkets making a virtue of necessity by refusing to handle some of the more suspect ones. There are signs of a new awareness, a movement towards making important social changes. We must put our shoulder to the wheel and add what push we can.

Recently someone at a table adjacent to mine in a small, crowded restaurant, took out a cigarette and waved it towards me before lighting it, saying, 'You don't mind do you . . .'. I don't know which of us was the more surprised when I said that I would rather he didn't smoke. I admit I found this quite difficult to do, but it gets easier every time. More and more people are turning their homes and offices into No Smoking zones and there are plenty of useful visual aids available to assist in this. My favourite is a little card on display in our local radiotherapy department that says 'Cancer Cures Smoking'.

The price of freedom is indeed constant vigilance. One good thing to come out of the accident at the Chernobyl nuclear power station is that it has aroused a keener sense of safety, and a greater awareness of possible risks, in nuclear stations all over the world. The other thing, perhaps even more important, is that we are aware now as perhaps never before that isolationist policies make no sense at all. What happened in Russia directly affected many other countries, and indirectly affected even more.

It has been brought home to us with shocking force that 'No man is an island entire of itself' and that 'Every man's death diminishes me, because I am involved in mankind'.

If forests in the northern hemisphere are being destroyed by acid rain then we should all check what we are pouring out of our factory chimneys and not sigh with relief because *our* forests are all right. I recently heard a doctor on the radio saying that she found it inconceivable that acid rain could affect trees and not humans.

It will be hard for some people to understand when I talk about things as different as nuclear radiation, E-numbers and emotional stress almost in the same sentence, and all in relation to cancer. Scientists talk about certain things being directly carcinogenic, other things being indirectly carcino-genic, and then they start muttering about co-agents. But classifying in this way is not as helpful as it might look at first.

The *Medical Encyclopedia* tells us 'By far the most signifi-cant chemical carcinogen is tobacco smoke'. So far so good: not smoking is something I can choose for myself, an area of my life where I can effect some control. But the fact that not everyone who smokes gets cancer, and that some smokers don't even get ill at all raises some questions. The Hunzas, that legendary race of healthy, happy people who seem to live for ever – they smoke, and cancer is almost unheard of amongst them. Time and again we come back to the fact that we cannot find a nice neat causative factor for cancer. We have to juggle with lots of different things at once. We have to think along much broader lines. Maybe the Hunzas, and others, can get away with smoking because they eat properly, their emotional needs are being met, and they are not bombarded by chemicals in the air they breathe and the water they drink. Whichever way we look we have to face the fact that man is polluting his planet and making it increasingly difficult for people to live healthy lives and avoid getting ill.

When cancer invades the body it behaves like a parasite. As it grows it demands more and more from us nutritionally and deposits more and more toxic matter into our body. It gives nothing back. It grows more and more demanding and greedy and flourishes at the expense of healthy tissues. In the end the parasite kills its host. Cancer both starves and poisons us to death.

Is this not exactly what we are doing to our planet, Earth? Man behaves in his world like a cancer. He leaches out more and more resources, replacing nothing. Not only is he greedy, he is also poisonous, disturbing the balance of the soil with dangerous chemicals, dumping piles of nuclear waste.

Years ago C. P. Snow said 'we shall watch them starve to death on television' and that is exactly what we are doing. Half the planet is starving and it would seem that the other half is being slowly poisoned. We could change this if we applied to our homes, our offices, our communities, our countries and our planet, the same holistic principles that we are applying to our bodies.

We need to practise a kind of ecological medicine. We must move towards a way of existing peacefully and uncompetitively with each other while we heal and restore our planet. Building the New Jerusalem can only be done through love, from the heart. It was Benjamin Disraeli who asked, 'Is man an ape or an angel?'

Like him, I am on the side of the angels. I believe we can do it.

Index

If you would like to purchase a copy of the tape referred to in this book (price £5. V.A.T. and p & p inclusive) please complete the following form.

To: Cancer Help Centre, Bristol
      Grove House
      Cornwallis Grove
      Clifton
      Bristol BS8 4PG
      (Tel. 0272 – 743216)

Please send .... copy/s of 'Helping with Healing'.

I enclose £............ cash/cheque/Barclaycard/Access/Visa

NAME: ....

Address ....

        ....

        ....

        ....

Signature ....

Access/Visa/Barclaycard No ....